Inspiring and Supporting Behavior Change

A Food and Nutrition Professional's Counseling Guide

Ann Constance, MA, RD, CDE,
AND Cecilia Sauter, MS, RD, CDE

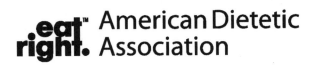

eat™ American Dietetic
right. Association

Diana Faulhaber, Publisher
Laura Pelehach, Acquisitions and Development Manager
Elizabeth Nishiura, Production Manager
Krisan Matthews, Assistant Development Editor

10 9 8 7 6 5 4 3 2 1

Library of Congress Cataloging-in-Publication Data

Constance, Ann.
  Inspiring and supporting behavior change : a food and nutrition professional's counseling guide / Ann Constance and Cecilia Sauter.
      p. ; cm.
  Includes bibliographical references and index.
  ISBN 978-0-88091-455-0
  1. Nutrition counseling.   2. Patient education.   3. Health promotion.
  I. Sauter, Cecilia.   II. American Dietetic Association.   III. Title.
  [DNLM: 1. Nutrition Therapy—methods. 2. Patient Education as Topic—methods.   3. Behavior Control—methods.   4. Diet.   5. Health Behavior.
  6. Health Promotion—methods. WB 400]
  RM218.7.C66 2011
  615.8′54—dc23

                                                                    2011022762

Contents

Contents

Chapter 7   When Patients Need More than
Nutrition Counseling 87

Chapter 8   Building Long-Term Support for Patients 105

Chapter 9   Other Issues to Consider:
Health Literacy, Cultural Diversity,
and Biases in Health Care 115

Appendix   Additional Resources 131

Acknowledgments

We appreciate and thank our husbands for supporting us as we wrote this book. They listened to our concerns, took over family and home responsibilities, and gave us the nudges we needed to keep on going.

Next we want to thank the editors at the American Dietetic Association who helped us fix grammatical errors and offered re-write suggestions to improve clarity and readability. Laura Pele-hach, Elizabeth Nishiura, and Krisan Matthews, you have been wonderful to work with. And a special thanks to the reviewers, Hope T. Bilyk, Marion J. Franz, Carol Grafford, Eileen S. Myers, Sandra A. Parker, and Julie Schwartz, who offered peer-to-peer critiques to help us improve this book.

We also have other special people in our lives who advised us on content and readability. Many, many thanks to Marti Funnell, MS, RN, CDE, an internationally recognized behavior change expert, for taking time to review our book, providing us with suggestions for improvement, sharing pertinent research articles with us, and writing the Foreword. Thanks to Rita Short, RD, for giving us valuable feedback, as a nutrition expert. In addition, we appreciate the detail-oriented family member, Beverly Teal, who offered many helpful suggestions on grammar and readability.

Reviewers

Hope T. Bilyk, MS, RD
North Chicago, Illinois

Marion J. Franz, MS, RD, CDE
Minneapolis, Minnesota

Carol Grafford, RD, CDE
Hancock, Michigan

Eileen S. Myers, MPH, RD, FADA
Nashville, Tennessee

Sandra A. Parker, RD, CDE
Walker, Michigan

Julie Schwartz, MS, RD, CSSD
Suwanee, Georgia

Foreword

Congratulations on choosing this book! I am honored to introduce you to this wonderful resource, which I know will be of help to your patients and to you as you implement these strategies and recommendations.

One of the most difficult things about working with chronically ill patients is dealing with behavior change. It is frustrating for us and frustrating for our patients. In spite of all of the information and good advice we give, our patients at times seem to ignore what we say and make choices that we know are not in the best interests of their long-term health.

In the past, many of our efforts were focused on helping patients be more compliant/adherent or on getting them to change. Health professionals often took credit for their patients' successes and blamed them for what we viewed as their failures. Many times, our attempts to get them to change only seemed to increase their resistance and created a negative cycle of our trying harder but patients becoming more and more resistant. In the worst cases, these patients were labeled as chronically noncompliant and we sometimes just gave up on them.

Fortunately, in recent years we have gained greater insights into working effectively with patients who have diabetes and other chronic illnesses. We have recognized that methods based on acute care models are not effective in treating chronic diseases, where most care is provided by patients and is, in fact, self-care or self-management. We now understand that our attempts to control patients' behaviors and decisions are ineffective. New models of care, such as the Chronic Care Model, and new strategies are needed to help patients manage the complexities of these illnesses on a daily basis. We need to help patients understand not only that they are in charge but also that they can *take* charge in ways that will work in the context of their lives, other priorities, and demands.

This understanding has come through insights gained from research in the area of diabetes-related distress, our own work in the area of patient empowerment, and the efforts of other behavioral scientists and clinicians working in the field. A great deal of effort in recent years has been devoted to creating patient-centered, collaborative models of care that focus on the needs of the patients and in better supporting their self-management efforts. Strategies such as meeting the patient's agenda during a visit; setting goals self-determined by the patient; helping patients feel more confident in their ability to make decisions, solve problems, and overcome barriers; and addressing the emotional side of diabetes have all been shown to be effective approaches to diabetes self-management. We also now know that, while providing education is effective, patients need ongoing self-management support to maintain behavior changes over a lifetime of chronic illness.

The key to implementing these strategies is to develop a partnership with our patients. In this partnership, the expertise of the patient is recognized as just as important as the expertise of the health professional. As health professionals, we acknowledge that, while we know about the clinical side of their illness, patients are the experts on their lives and what will work for them. They know what they have tried in the past that has and has not worked, the barriers they will face, the support that is available to them, and the competing demands and priorities they juggle each day. We also need to help them understand how diabetes-related distress—the everyday anger, fear, frustration, and guilt most patients experience—influences their behavior. In short, our interactions need to encompass all of these aspects of diabetes (or other chronic disease) if our patients' self-management efforts are to be successful.

We also need to help our patients understand that many of our efforts, and many of their own, will be trial and error. These "experiments" are not failures on our part or theirs. They are simply among the realities of a chronic disease, particularly ones as complex as diabetes. The goal is to keep trying until together we find the plan that works for their illness and, just as importantly, for their lives.

This book will help you put all of this together in a practical way as you work with patients. Ann and Cecilia have created a great resource because it provides a great deal of information about how to help patients who are interested in making lifestyle changes and how various approaches will work in different situations. In short, this book gives you the tools you need to be an effective registered dietitian as you work with patients who have diabetes or another chronic condition.

A key theme for the National Diabetes Education Program (NDEP) over the past 2 years has been, "Managing diabetes. It's not easy, but it's worth it." This is the message that we need to convey to our patients. With our help through the strategies delineated in this book, they can do it!

Martha M. Funnell, MS, RN, CDE
Research Investigator
Department of Medical Education
University of Michigan Medical School
Ann Arbor, MI

Preface

Through our work experiences, additional training, and influence of our mentors, we have confirmed that our approach to working with patients is critical to their success in making lifestyle changes. While our clinical skills and expertise as food and nutrition professionals are important, they mean little if we don't connect with people in a way that inspires them to want to change. Our goal in this book is to give you an overview of the most commonly used approaches to guide patients through lifestyle changes. We provide reinforcement for these approaches through scenarios and practice exercises.

There are many reasons why patients may be labeled as "noncompliant." We have learned that patients often need to work on other issues before they can successfully make lifestyle changes. In this book, we provide tools to help you identify and deal with many of those concerns, like depression, health distress, and low health literacy. By using these tools, you can help improve patient success. In addition, we discuss the importance of providing patients with ongoing support from clinicians, family, community services, and/or Internet resources. These are among the keys to effectively helping our patients live healthier lives.

We decided to write this book to reinforce the importance of a food and nutrition professional's counseling skills and approach to patient care. While much of your dietetics education up to this point has likely focused on important nutrition topics and interventions, this book is meant to deepen your abilities to inspire and motivate your patients. It can help you move your patients to the point where they are ready to hear about nutrition interventions and can effectively put their newfound knowledge into practice.

We hope this book will help you become a more effective clinician, which translates into healthier and happier patients. In turn, your patients' success will foster an enhanced sense of job satisfaction.

Ann Constance, MA, RD, CDE
Cecilia Sauter, MS, RD, CDE

1

Oh, No! Don't Tell Me I Have to Change!

Nobody likes change except a baby in wet diapers.

In a perfect world, our patients would always be motivated to follow our recommendations. Once they leave our offices, they would immediately implement the meal plan ideas we presented. They'd start being more physically active. They'd even start eating whole grains! As they moved toward their health goals, they would begin seeing results and, before long, they'd send us bouquets of "thank you" flowers. Of course, we live in the real world, and we know that human behavior is more complex than that.

Bob's Story

Take Bob, for example. Bob is 65 years old, has poorly controlled type 2 diabetes, and weighs almost 300 pounds. In addition, his blood pressure, cholesterol, and triglycerides are too high, his HDL cholesterol is only 28 mg/dL, and he is taking several

1

medications. Bob's doctor referred him to a registered dietitian (RD), Susan, to help learn how to make changes to his eating habits, which will assist with weight loss and getting his blood glucose under better control.

At Bob's first appointment, Susan weighs and measures him. She also asks several questions about his current level of physical activity and how often he eats out each week. Then she calculates the number of calories Bob needs to consume each day to begin losing weight slowly (1 to 2 pounds per week) and develops a meal plan for him based on that number. For the remainder of the appointment, Susan and Bob go over the suggested meal plan, and Susan offers plenty of advice about what to eat. She uses food models to teach Bob about portion control. She also gives Bob a comprehensive "eating out" handout to take home. If he follows these instructions, he should begin to see results!

Bob never follows the great advice from this trained nutrition expert. He is used to skipping breakfast, often missing lunch, and then eating a big dinner and grazing for the rest of the evening. In contrast, Susan designed a plan that included three meals and an evening snack each day. To Bob, this meal plan seems overwhelming and unacceptable. He feels like he's being asked to make many changes at once, and most of the changes involve things he has been doing for many years. In addition, he does not really see the benefit in making these changes. As is too often the case in the health care arena, Bob fails to keep his follow-up appointment with Susan.

Reaching the "Unreachable" Patient

What went wrong? Are patients like Bob "unreachable"? Are they destined for the noncompliant/no-show section of our file drawer or for the "inactive patients" file in our computer database? Could

Susan the RD have done things differently to help Bob identify changes he was willing to make and follow through with?

How many of your patients secretly dread that you are going to make them stop eating all of their favorite foods? How many splurge the day or week before seeing you, anticipating that their favorite foods will soon be "forbidden"? How many think they will have to give up foods that taste good, because the foods cannot be healthy for them? Perhaps they expect they will be eating nothing but lettuce, broccoli, and high-fiber cereal for the rest of their lives. Whether your patients have diabetes, kidney disease, obesity, or any number of other health conditions, these thoughts are probably going through their minds.

We know nutrition and exercise are just as important as medication to improve or maintain health, but many patients find changes to their food and activity habits much more difficult than taking medication. And, frankly, they may not *want* to change, or they may not realize how crucial these modifications are to their health.

RDs face such challenges every day. That's why we wrote this book—to give you the tools and know-how to inspire patients to take control and manage lifestyle changes for better health. In addition to your clinical knowledge, you can learn to become an effective change agent!

Success Is All in the Approach

"It is not necessary to change. Survival is not mandatory."
—W. Edwards Deming

How we approach and support our patients can be critical to whether or not they successfully make difficult lifestyle changes. As a trained food and nutrition expert, you have a lot of great advice to share with your patients. What you may need to learn is *how* and *when* to share that expertise. If knowledge was the single most important thing we needed to share with patients, we would have thousands of reformed eaters in our communities. Our friends, family members, and co-workers would be "perfect eaters" too! In addition, no one would smoke, and all of us would get at least 120 minutes of physical activity each week!

In Bob's case, he received enough education. Susan certainly gave him the *information* he needed to make lifestyle changes. Bob, however, lacked the *desire* to change and *confidence* to follow through on the proposed changes.

In this book, we will teach you how to be more successful when counseling patients. We will discuss ways to help patients identify what is most important to them, to work with them to set goals, and to enhance their confidence in making the changes. We will show you how to wrap-up patient visits by collaborating to make a plan that is important to them and one they think they can complete over the course of the next week or two.

The process of figuring out what the patient really wants and feels willing to do might take skills you haven't fully developed in the classroom or continuing education programs. In this book, you will learn ways to identify a patient's willingness to change. We will also show you how to use strategies like motivational interviewing to help guide patients toward making their own behavior change plans, which they will be more likely to implement.

We discuss how to form partnerships with patients and help empower them to take charge of their lives and lifestyle changes. We explain how to help patients look at their options for change as well as the consequences of not making these adjustments. And we demonstrate the value of supporting patients in making small improvements as well as large ones—over time, baby steps can add up to a *big* change!

Reading this book can also help you hone your listening skills. We discuss communication techniques, like reflective listening, that will enhance your patients' willingness to change.

Paul's Story: Similar Situation, Different Result

"Insanity: Doing the same thing over and over again and expecting different results."
—ALBERT EINSTEIN

If your patients are not making changes or are not coming back for follow-up appointments, perhaps it is time for *you* to try a different approach. In that light, let's turn to Paul's story.

Paul is an avid hunter in the Upper Peninsula of Michigan, who shares many of the same health concerns as Bob. He is in his sixties, has had poorly controlled diabetes for many years, and, like Bob, is overweight, has elevated blood pressure and abnormal lipids, and takes many medications. Paul also recently had coronary bypass surgery. Unfortunately, the incision on his lower leg is not healing, and he is at risk for having his leg amputated.

The opening day of deer hunting season is coming up. Paul looks forward to meeting his friends at hunting camp every year. He is motivated to do anything to save his leg and make it to hunting camp this year. Taking his doctor's advice, Paul makes an appointment with an RD, Irene, for medical nutrition therapy.

During the first encounter, Irene spends time getting to know Paul in order to understand what is important to him. She asks why he came for nutrition counseling today and what his greatest concern is. Paul replies that he wants his leg to heal so he can hunt. Their conversation then turns to what Paul already knows about diabetes, controlling diabetes, and how diabetes is linked to wound healing. Guided by pertinent questions from Irene,

Paul identifies a couple of changes he is willing to make while still keeping his focus on the prize—going to hunting camp.

Irene recognizes that Paul needs to decide what *he* wants to work on and helps him set a goal to accomplish over the next 1 to 2 weeks. Before the session ends, Irene checks to make sure that Paul has a high level of confidence to follow through on the action steps he set for himself. Luckily, Paul has also brought a support person to the visit, his wife, Jan. Her participation is important because she does most of the grocery shopping and cooking. Over the next couple of weeks, Paul is indeed motivated to take action, and his blood glucose levels improve. He returns for his follow up appointments, too. If his health continues to improve, he can focus on what he truly enjoys—his hunting trips.

It should be clear why Paul was able to meet his goals but Bob wasn't. In Paul's case, Irene the RD focused on his motivations for seeking medical nutrition therapy. In Bob's case, Susan the RD never found out much about him, his likes and interests, or his motivations. She also didn't find out what Bob already knew about diabetes. Susan directed their conversation and presented him with changes to make, rather than involving Bob in the process.

Forming Relationships

As the stories of Bob and Paul illustrate, developing rapport is key when working with patients. However, for some RDs, the ability to form relationships may not come naturally. It might help to think of your role as that of a salesperson. Successful salespeople listen to what people want and build trust with their customers. You can use similar techniques to identify patient concerns and priorities during nutrition counseling. The successful "sale" for the RD comes when the patient sets a goal and achieves it!

What's Next?

This book focuses primarily on the work you do with your patients on an individual basis. However, your patients may also have a difficult time making and sustaining behavior change because the health system is not set up to effectively help patients with chronic health care conditions. Chapter 2 therefore discusses some of the challenges that you and your patients may encounter in the health care system and in the community, as well as solutions that institutions, communities, and individual RDs can seek.

In Chapters 3 through 6, you will find tips and techniques for helping patients identify what is most important to them regarding health goals. More specifically, Chapter 3 looks at empowering patients; Chapter 4 covers the stages of change model of behavior change; and Chapter 5 explains motivational interviewing. In Chapter 6, we put these strategies together as we guide you through processes that will help you assist your patients to set reasonable, self-selected goals—goals they will take ownership of, not react to.

Throughout this book, you'll find examples of how emotions can affect patients' desire and ability to change. One of the authors of this book met a man with diabetes who compared his experiences of living with diabetes to when he was diagnosed with and treated for colon cancer. He said the negative emotions associated with diabetes management were *more* pronounced than the negative emotions surrounding his cancer diagnosis and treatment. During his cancer treatment, this man had a fairly passive role—once the appropriate treatment was determined, he just "sat back" and let the health care professionals perform surgery and administer chemotherapy. At every visit related to his cancer treatment, the medical staff checked on his mental and emotional health, too. With diabetes, *he* had to make and carry out most of the decisions—what to eat, how much insulin to take, when to check his blood glucose, and what to do if his glucose levels went too high or too low (1). Unfortunately, his diabetes care providers did not check on or provide assistance for diabetes distress or anxiety. Chapter 7 explores further the effect of diabetes distress and offers advice about working with patients who may need emotional or mental health support as well as treatment for serious health problems. The chapter addresses ways to identify patients who may have emotional/mental health issues like anxiety and depression, and how to refer them for additional care when their needs go beyond the scope of your practice. This chapter also includes guidance on financial resources for patients whose adherence with treatment may be affected by economic constraints.

In Chapter 8, we discuss the topic of building long-term support for behavior change. Options for professional and peer support are surveyed. Chapter 9 examines a number of communication-related issues that can affect your counseling abilities—health literacy of patients, cultural and ethnic diversity, and a variety of potential biases that may shape your perspective. The book also includes an appendix of resources for RDs seeking further information.

When you inspire and support behavior change, you set up a win-win-win situation. First, patients feel good when they are successful. Also, you are excited about no longer being the "bad guy" or feeling that you bear most of the responsibility for patient change—change is in the hands of each patient, and they are setting and accomplishing their health behavior goals. Finally, the health care provider loves seeing health improvements, especially in patients who were once labeled as being noncompliant or resistant to change.

Practice Exercises

Exercise 1

Think about your patients and ask yourself the following questions:

- What percentage of your patients comes back for follow-up care?
- How many patients are setting and achieving goals? How many are also improving health parameters?
- How many of your patients would you label as "noncompliant"?

Exercise 2

Now, think about yourself and your own personal health habits and answer the following questions:

- Have you been thinking about changing any of your own health habits?
- Have you taken action on these changes?
- If so, have you been successful? What helped you make the changes?
- If not, why not? What are the barriers you are facing?

Reference

1. Weiss MA, Funnell MM. *The Little Diabetes Book You Need to Read.* Philadelphia, PA: Running Press; 2007.

2

Patients Change . . . When *We* Change: The Chronic Care Model

"Everyone thinks of changing the world,
but no one thinks of changing himself."

—LEO TOLSTOY

In Chapter 1 we introduced you to Bob and Paul, two men with similar health challenges, including diabetes and overweight, who responded very differently to their encounters with registered dietitians (RDs). Bob disregarded the advice of his RD and never returned for follow-up. In contrast, Paul succeeded in making changes and demonstrated a willingness to engage in follow-up nutrition counseling. As we sought to explain the different outcomes, we attributed Paul's greater success to the approach his RD used, which emphasized listening to his needs and interests and helping him set goals based on his personal priorities, such as his desire to go to hunting camp.

Neither of these stories mentioned the training or resources available to the RDs, the health care systems in which they worked, or the characteristics of the surrounding communities. How might these sorts of factors contribute to the opportunities for patients to achieve personal success? That question is addressed in this chapter. In particular, we examine the distinctions between acute and chronic health care and explore the components of a model of health care focused on the management of chronic health conditions. As we shall show, system-wide implementation of this Chronic Care Model (CCM) can support the individual efforts of RDs and other clinicians to improve patient outcomes.

The Scope of Chronic Health Care Demands

Historically, the health care system in the United States was set up to primarily treat *acute* (short-duration) medical problems. For example, a patient would visit a physician when he or she had an illness like pneumonia or an injury like a broken leg. In those cases, the physician was regarded as the expert and the patient's role was limited and mostly passive, relying on the recommendations of the doctor.

Today, many patient visits to the health care provider are related to *chronic* conditions, such as diabetes, heart disease, or arthritis. According to estimates from the Institute of Medicine (1), 134 million Americans will have a chronic condition in 2020. Other sources estimate that 80% of outpatient care is linked to providing support for chronic or lifelong illnesses like type 1 and type 2 diabetes, obesity, or heart disease (2). In 2005 the United States spent $2 trillion on health care, and chronic illness accounted for 75% of the spending (3). In the Medicare program, 96% of expenditures were for chronic conditions (4).

Supporting Self-Management

"The name of the game is taking care of yourself because you're going to live long enough to wish you had."
—Grace Mirabella

In contrast to traditional administration of acute medical care, most care for chronic disease is usually done by the patient between appointments (self-management) while the health care provider's role has shifted to a more passive one, similar to that of a coach or adviser (5). The reality of a chronic disease is that the patient has the right and the responsibility to make self-management decisions on a daily basis. As Bodenheimer and associates explain (6):

> *Self-management* is what people do every day: they decide what to eat, whether or not to exercise, if and when they will monitor their health, or whether or not they will take their medications. Everyone self-manages, even the patient who chooses *not* to take care of himself. So the question becomes whether or not the choices made will improve their health-related behaviors and therefore lead them to improve their clinical outcomes.

Unfortunately, while the demands of chronic diseases on the health care system have increased greatly, the training of many health care professionals is still based on the older paradigm of dealing with acute illness, where active patient participation is less important. In general, health care providers have not been adequately prepared to deal with chronic conditions, and many health care and community organizations lack systems and programs to treat and support people with chronic health issues (7,8). Adopting strategies to support the self-management efforts of our patients will enhance our interactions with them and minimize everyone's frustration.

There are three fundamental aspects of chronic care: choices, control, and consequences. Patients make choices every day, and these choices have a greater impact on their health than the recommendations of health care providers. Also, patients are in charge of their own lives. They decide which recommendations they will follow and which ones they will ignore. Finally, because patients are the ones who make the decisions that best fit into their lives, they are also responsible for the consequences of their decisions (7,9,10). Many of us may have to fight the urge to try to "fix" our patients—after all, we have so much knowledge and advice to offer that we know our patients would benefit from following!

Self-management in chronic disease usually requires multiple lifestyle changes. However, many health care providers believe they know best which changes the patient needs to make, and they therefore tell the patient how, where, and when to make these lifestyle changes. These providers believe that their expertise in the treatment of the disease also makes them the "expert" of what changes will help the patient the most, regardless of the patient's desires or interests. However, when we ignore or downplay our patients' concerns and priorities, they feel our recommendations are intrusive, and they may not be ready or able to follow our advice. This can also lead to providers feeling frustrated because they cannot get their patients to follow their recommendations. These patients are often called "noncompliant" (10).

Studies have demonstrated that patients often don't follow the advice and recommendations of clinicians. As many as 50% of patients don't follow long-term medication regimens, more than

80% don't follow advice to change health behaviors, and 20% to 30% don't complete curative medication regimens (11,12). These statistics may be startling, but they indicate that we need to look at different ways to help our patients help themselves!

When we use good communication skills, more patients are able to follow our recommendations and improve self-care. In these situations, patients are more satisfied with their care and have better health outcomes. In short, to improve outcomes, we must collaborate with patients and encourage their participation in treatment decisions (13). As an RD, you are the expert in nutrition, but your patients are the experts in knowing what does and what does not work for them and what they are willing to try.

The Chronic Care Model

As an individual RD, you can do a great deal to strengthen your counseling skills to inspire and support behavior change by your patients (see Chapters 3 through 9). Identifying ways to improve care of patients with chronic conditions may enhance your opportunities for success, and the Chronic Care Model (CCM) is one option your health system may want to explore.

The Chronic Care Model focuses on strengthening chronic illness management within the primary care setting. Dr. Ed Wagner and his team at the MacColl Institute at Group Health Cooperative in Seattle, with funding from the Robert Wood Johnson Foundation, developed the CCM. This model places the responsibility for self-management with the affected individual, while also emphasizing the importance of structured self-management support activities and systems within communities to facilitate healthy behavior changes (see Figure 2.1) (14).

According to the CCM, health outcomes improve when the informed and activated patient works with a health care team that

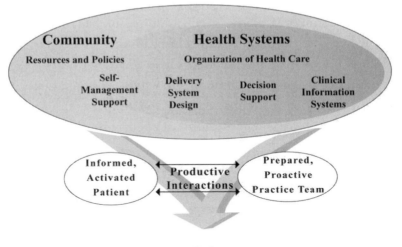

Improved Outcomes

FIGURE 2.1 The Chronic Care Model. Reprinted with permission from Wagner EH. Chronic disease management: what will it take to improve care for chronic illness? *Eff Clin Pract.* 1998;1:2–4.

is prepared and trained to be proactive and collaborative (8). The patient and clinicians are both important parts of the CCM. Thus, the double arrows between the patient and clinicians in Figure 2.1 suggest the reciprocal nature of their interaction. An empowered and activated patient may stimulate the clinician to move into action in a partnership type of a relationship, while clinicians (including RDs) who are trained to be patient centered and collaborative are more likely to empower and engage their patients.

In addition to the patient and his or her team of health care providers, the health care system is a large component of the CCM (see Figure 2.1). Advocates of this model seek to create a culture within health care delivery organizations that prioritizes chronic care, as well as the necessary mechanisms to promote safe and high-quality care for patients.

Clearly, RDs play a role in this part of the CCM. Even if you are in private practice, you must often coordinate patient care with other team members associated with one or more health care systems. For example, your ability to provide optimal care depends on a health care system that allows you to do the following:

- Identify patients who have not received their routine care or have missed their follow-up appointments with other members of the health care team.
- Access patients' health parameters (such as laboratory test results, data from examinations, and health status) that are relevant to the scope of practice of the RD.

The final component of the CCM is the community. Forming partnerships between health care systems and organizations that offer community resources enhances patient support. Some community organizations are also instrumental in developing interventions that will fill the gaps in health care services. RDs can be key players in directing patients to effective community programs (14). In addition, RDs can promote the adoption of public policies that support healthful living, such as smoke-free public areas and walkable communities. As you work with patients, you must know of, and perhaps even assist with, the development of community programs and policies that support your patients. You will find more details about self-management support through community resources and technology in Chapters 7 and 8.

Health Care Systems and Chronic Care

To effectively treat patients with chronic health conditions, certain aspects of the health care system need to be oriented toward chronic care: the clinician information system, decision support, delivery system design, and self-management support.

Clinician Information System

A clinician information system organizes patient data to facilitate efficient and effective care. For example, a registry of all the patients who have diabetes within an institution helps to track their care and outcomes. Such a registry facilitates the planning of the individual patient care and makes it possible to share information with patients and providers, coordinate care, and improve outcomes. How does this benefit the RD? The registry could identify patients who would benefit from medical nutrition therapy, and their records could be flagged to ensure they receive a referral to an RD.

Decision Support

Decision support refers to information that promotes clinician care that is consistent with scientific evidence and patient preferences. Decision support integrates evidence-based guidelines with daily clinical practice, making it possible to share evidence-based information with patients, which may encourage their participation in self-care. For instance, when you explain the "ABCs" of diabetes care (ie, A1c; blood pressure; cholesterol control) to a patient and provide information about how to attain those goals, you can help her become more proactive in her own care. As a result, she will know what the desirable health goals are and be aware of the changes needed to attain those goals.

Using evidence-based care also helps all members of the health care team stay on the same track. For example, a doctor who writes orders for a 1,000- or 1,200 calorie diet for *all* patients with diabetes is not practicing evidence-based or patient-centered care. In fact, practices like this can be counterproductive and unreasonable, resulting in patients giving up on making changes because the recommendations are too onerous. Such patients may never return to you for follow-up and may limit their visits to other providers as well. In such situations, patients may not feel better and may be at higher risk for complications if they do not seek medical care. Then the health care system (and taxpayers) must take care of costly complications, many of which could have been prevented through good self-care. Finally, the health care provider is affected with concern and frustration for patients who are "noncompliant."

Delivery System Design

A well-designed delivery system ensures that patients receive effective, efficient clinical care, as well as appropriate self-management support. It is critical that the design consider health literacy and cultural sensitivity (see Chapter 9). Within this system, we can include planned patient visits or group visits for diabetes or other chronic health conditions, as well as clinical case management services for patients with complex health issues. An appropriate health care delivery system will refer patients to RDs for care or follow-up. As an RD, you can assist with care management, too.

Self-Management Support

Self-management support empowers and prepares patients to manage their health and care. Effective self-management support strategies include appropriate assessment, setting goals, action planning, problem solving and follow up. You cannot possibly be the sole or main support person or resource for all of your patients. Seek out internal and community resources that will provide ongoing self-management support to patients. Help link them to the type of support that works best for them. These efforts will also enhance patient success.

Implementing the Chronic Care Model

"All governments must be prepared to deal with the infectious diseases because they could be overwhelming this year or next, but the long-term problem is with the chronic diseases."
—ROBERT BEAGLEHOLE,
Director of the Department of Chronic Disease
and Health Promotion,
World Health Organization, 2003–2007

The CCM is an evidence-based approach. When all or some of the components are implemented, the model supports your patients in setting and achieving their goals. Let us therefore explore how to implement the CCM within health care institutions.

According to the Institute of Medicine (1), multiple changes are needed to make our health care system support chronic care management. Detailed information about how health care systems can enhance chronic care management is available on the Making System Changes for Better Diabetes Care Web site (15). RDs employed by health care organizations may be part of chronic care management teams and can also play a role in system redesign. This Web site offers resources that can help with needed system changes.

You can help to implement evidence-based care in your health care system. When all team members and patients share a consistent approach and objectives, patients are less confused (15). Look for opportunities to be part of guideline implementation teams for your health care system, especially for guidelines linked to the RD scope of practice. For example, some health care systems may use electronic health records with embedded clinical guidelines, and perhaps you can help review or adapt these guidelines to fit the needs of the organization. Other health care systems may need to go through a formal process to develop, implement, and review guidelines that are evidence based and will be used by all health care team members. You may be able to participate in the following parts of the process:

- Putting together a guideline development team
- Looking at existing evidence—guidelines already in place and recent research on the issue
- Customizing guidelines based on research and the needs of a particular facility
- Identifying ways to integrate guideline use
- Assessing guideline use
- Planning regular reviews and revisions

Ideally, once guidelines are developed, they are supported by automated clinical information and decision support systems through electronic health records. With electronic health records, you can access evidence-based guidelines that other team members use in patient treatment. When appropriate, you can then help reinforce guidelines with patient and/or contact another provider when additional care is indicated. For example, if you note that a patient with diabetes has not had a dilated eye exam in more than a year, you could explore that with him. Perhaps he is unaware of the guidelines for eye exams in diabetes care, or he might face other barriers to eye care that the health care team has not addressed.

Similarly, the electronic health record can also identify for other team members the latest and greatest findings on nutrition interventions. For example, as RDs, we know that there is no "one size fits all" diet for people with diabetes. With our patients, we collaboratively develop personalized meal plans based on patient goals, preferences, glucose control, and other comorbidities. When the evidence-based guidelines for diabetes meal planning are disseminated to other health care professionals, they can reinforce the recommendations and diminish the use of fad diets. Therefore, RDs should be involved in guideline development for health care systems or participate in the review of guidelines already implemented.

In addition to participating in the integration of evidence-based guidelines into your health care system, you can also improve chronic care by advocating for systemic support for patient-centered care. See Table 2.1 for the "new rules" of this type of care (1). Well-planned communication channels through regular team meetings and information technology are one essential step, as it is critical to coordinate patient care in various settings over time.

As you counsel patients, you will want to adjust your approach based on their personal ability to set and achieve goals, but you will also want to consider the structure of the health care system, as well as the availability of other support systems within the community and in the health care system. This process is a bit like juggling several balls at once. It involves more than just working with patients; you also help implement the recommendations of the CCM on a system- and community-wide basis.

TABLE 2.1 *Rules for Effective Health Care*

New Rule	Current Rule
Care is based on continuous healing relationships.	Care is based primarily on visits.
Care is customized according to patients' needs and values.	Professional autonomy drives variability.
The patient is the source of control.	Professionals control care.
Knowledge is shared freely.	Information is a record.
Decision-making is based on evidence.	Decision-making is based on training and experience.
Safety is a system property.	"Do no harm" is an individual responsibility.
Transparency is necessary.	Secrecy is necessary.
Needs are anticipated.	The system reacts to needs.
Waste is continuously decreased.	Cost reduction is sought.
Cooperation among clinicians is a priority.	Preference is given to professional roles over the system.

Source: Reprinted with permission from Committee on Quality of Health Care in America, Institute of Medicine. *Crossing the Quality Chasm: A New Health System for the 21st Century.* Washington, DC: National Academies Press; 2001:61–62.

Practice Exercises

Exercise 1

List the various health care system or community resources you currently coordinate patient care with. Are there any types of resources that are needed?

Exercise 2

If you work with or in a health care system, are there parts of the Chronic Care Model that are not already in place that you can help implement? If so, what are they and what steps will you take to make these changes?

References

1. Committee on Quality of Health Care in America, Institute of Medicine. *Crossing the Quality Chasm: A New Health System for the 21st Century.* Washington, DC: National Academies Press; 2001. http://books .nap.edu/openbook.php?record_id=10027. Accessed December 7, 2009.

2. Grumbach K, Bodenheimer T. A primary care home for Americans: putting the house in order. *JAMA.* 2002;288:889–893

3. Centers for Disease Control and Prevention. Chronic Disease Prevention and Health Promotion. http://www.cdc.gov/nccdphp/overview .htm. Accessed February 24, 2010.

4. Partnership for Solutions. Chronic Conditions: Making the Case for Ongoing Care. September 2004 Update. http://www.rwjf.org/files/ research/Chronic%20Conditions%20Chartbook%209-2004.ppt. Accessed February 24, 2010.

5. Heisler M. Helping your patient with chronic disease: effective physician approaches to support self-management. *Semin Med Pract.* 2005;8:43–54.

6. Bodenheimer T, MacGregor K, Sharifi C. Helping patients manage their chronic conditions. 2005. California Healthcare Foundation. http://www.chcf.org/publications/2005/06/helping-patients-manage-their-chronic-conditions. Accessed December 2, 2009.

7. Funnell M, Anderson R. Empowerment and self-management of diabetes. *Clin Diabetes.* 2004;22:123–127.

8. Bodenheimer T, Loring K, Holman H, Grumbach K. Patient self-management of chronic disease in primary care. *JAMA.* 2002;288:2469–2475.

9. Glasgow RE, Anderson RM. In diabetes care, moving from compliance to adherence is not enough: something entirely different is needed [letter]. *Diabetes Care.* 1999;22:2090–2092.

10. Rubin RR, Anderson RM, Funnell MM. Collaborative diabetes care. *Pract Diabetol.* 2002;21:29–32.

11. Meichenbaum D, Turk DC. *Facilitating Treatment Adherence: A Practitioner's Guidebook.* New York, NY: Plenum; 1987.

12. DiMatteo MR. Enhancing patient adherence to medical recommendations. *JAMA.* 1994;271:29.

13. Funnell MM, Anderson RM. The problem with compliance in diabetes. *JAMA.* 2000;284:1709.

14. Wagner EH. Chronic disease management: what will it take to improve care for chronic illness? *Eff Clin Pract.* 1998;1:2–4.

15. National Diabetes Education Program, National Institutes of Health. Making Systems Changes for Better Diabetes Care. http://betterdiabetescare.nih.gov. Accessed December 7, 2009.

3

Empowerment: Putting Your Patients in the Driver's Seat

As we discussed in Chapter 2, the choices that patients make every day will have a much larger impact on chronic disease outcomes than any decision the health care providers make during the medical appointments (1–3). Patients' choices will affect how they live. Therefore, patients are responsible not only for their decisions but also for managing their disease (1–3). The challenge for registered dietitians (RDs) and other health care professionals is to provide care that empowers patients to make choices and follow through on behavior change. In that light, let's consider Jeff and Ana's stories.

Jeff's Story: Part 1

Jeff is the CEO of a large corporation. He gets his annual health exam at one of the most renowned clinics in the area. During his most recent exam, he was told that his blood pressure was elevated and he also has diabetes. Jeff met with a nurse who explained how to monitor his blood glucose and with an RD who provided instruction on how to modify his diet and lose weight. In addition, he received prescriptions for blood pressure and diabetes medications.

Jeff found it difficult to comply with all aspects of his care. In his work life, he had many meetings and ate out quite often. He found it hard to watch what he was eating. What's more, he often forgot to take his pills, and his busy job also kept him from going to the gym. When he finally went back to see his doctor, he had gained weight, his A1c had increased by 2%, and his blood pressure was still elevated.

Ana's Story

Ana is a hair stylist who has been feeling very tired lately. She does not have health insurance. When she found out that a health fair in town was offering health screenings, she decided to go. At the health fair, she learned her blood glucose was elevated and she most likely has diabetes. Ana decided to see a doctor at a small clinic close to her work. Since the clinic offered sliding-scale fees for office visits and medications, Ana was able to fit her care into her budget. At her first appointment, the doctor asked her the reason for her visit and what she was hoping to get out of the visit. Ana explained the results of her screening and that she wanted to learn more about diabetes, especially how to manage it. After confirming a diabetes diagnosis, the doctor explained to Ana that her A1c was 10% and medication would help her control diabetes. He also explained that lifestyle changes would be very helpful and asked whether she would be willing to meet with an RD for nutrition counseling. Ana agreed to schedule an appointment with the RD, Marissa.

During their first meeting, Marissa asked Ana what she already knew about diabetes and how to manage it, as well as how she felt about the diagnosis. As she found out more about Ana, Marissa offered some strategies Ana could choose that might fit into her lifestyle. With guidance from Marissa (who mainly asked questions), Ana chose a goal she believed to be a realistic starting point. Ana decided she would incorporate walking into her daily routine, and she and Marissa explored ideas for how she would accomplish this. Marissa reinforced how physical activity can positively affect Ana's blood glucose and overall health. Marissa also asked Ana whether she would like more resources to look over. Based on Ana's preferences, Marissa gave Ana a list of helpful Web sites and books. Marissa also provided information to Ana about low-cost and free community resources.

Ana joined a weight loss group and started walking most days of the week. Follow-up with Marissa and reading books about diabetes helped Ana to also change her cooking style and start eating smaller portions. By the time she returned 3 months later to see her doctor, Ana had lost weight and her A1c had decreased to 7.8%. Plus, Ana reported that she had a lot more energy.

Comparing Ana and Jeff's Stories

What is the difference between Ana's story and Jeff's? Is Ana more motivated than Jeff? Or is something else at work here?

Let's look first at Jeff's situation. The fact that he went to a renowned clinic where he received care from a group of medical experts did not improve his outcome. From the description of the encounter, it seems like Jeff did not have much of a role in developing the plan that he was responsible for implementing. The clinic he visited followed the "traditional" model of care, in which the health care professional is the authority responsible for the diagnosis and treatment as well as for the outcomes. In this model, patient education is generally prescriptive rather than collaborative. The health care professionals tell the patient what to do and set the goals for the patient. In Jeff's case, he was told to change his diet, exercise, and lose weight. Nobody asked him what he wanted to do or how he wanted to approach his care. The health care team did not take his busy lifestyle into consideration. The assumption was that Jeff is obligated to follow the advice of the health care professionals he saw. Since Jeff did not follow the recommendations the experts gave him, he was labeled "noncompliant."

How about Ana? She went to a small clinic—not the prestigious facility visited by Jeff. However, she succeeded in taking charge of her health outcomes. From the first interaction with a heath care professional, she was asked the reason for her visit and what she was hoping to get out of this visit. The physician asked for Ana's agenda and did not impose his own. The RD, Marissa, also asked Ana what she wanted to change and what she could reasonably achieve. Ana was part of the team. She worked *with* her health care providers instead of just following *their* directions. She set her own goals, and Marissa guided her to additional resources and information for managing diabetes. Marissa also helped Ana identify community-based support to help her in the future. What really makes the difference is listening to patients and involving them in their care.

As Jeff and Ana's stories demonstrate, your work with patients will be more effective when you make sure that their self-management plans fit their specific goals and takes into consideration their particular lifestyle and culture (for more details about cultural issues, refer to Chapter 9). Patients, not health care providers, set the goals. When patients choose their own goals, they will be more apt to stick with them and do the work needed to achieve them. The goals will also fit their lifestyles better, because patients know what works and does not work for them.

To help our patients, it is important that we learn to work *with* our patients. One way of working with our patients is to use the empowerment approach.

The Empowerment Approach

Patient empowerment is defined as "helping patients discover and develop the inherent capacity to be responsible for one's own life" (4). The empowerment approach is not just another tool we pull out of our kit when we are trying to help our patients to be more motivated and engaged. Empowerment is more of a philosophy in which the patient and the health care provider have their own roles. You will want to clarify these roles during your first encounter with a patient. From the start of care, empowered patients play an active role. They give you feedback regarding what works and what does not work, and they tell you what their biggest concerns are. On the other hand, you are available to help and assist patients in the process. You partner with patients to help them choose goals and create action plans, and you help identify barriers to change as well as strategies to overcome them. You also collaborate with patients by providing care recommendations, expert advice, and support. As Funnell and colleagues stated, "Professionals need to give up feeling responsible *for* their patients and become responsible *to* them" (2).

In the traditional approach, clinicians provide education based on what *they* believe the patient needs to know. In the empowerment approach, the patient asks questions and you provide the education that responds to these questions. You base education on the needs of the particular patient and do not provide instructions simply as part of "standard" care (2). The patient has a choice in deciding what information he needs to know so he can make better decisions related to his health. Of course, in some cases, a patient may not be sure what she wants to ask—in such instances, you may offer some suggestions of topics that may be appropriate to discuss based on where the patient is currently in her disease process. Patients are also able to set the agenda to make sure their concerns and needs are being addressed (2).

In Ana's case, she learned about diabetes, her treatment options, and strategies. The education, however, was based on what she needed to know right now—not what might benefit her in 10 years. She did not learn about every medication on the market for diabetes. She only learned about the specific medication that she was going to take and how it would affect her daily life. Her education also focused on the lifestyle changes that she was able to make at this point in time. Because Ana could use the information right away, she knew what to expect and could better determine whether the medication was really making a difference in her diabetes as well as what impact the exercise had on her blood glucose. Giving patients the tools to be proactive is the main goal of the empowerment approach. Ana got the tools she needed to start taking care of her diabetes based on her current needs, desires, and cultural background. She also received access to resources so she could continue exploring other possible approaches. Finally, yet most importantly, Ana and her RD worked together to create a goal and a plan.

Goal Setting

Goal setting is a very important part of the empowerment approach. The goal is a guide that helps each patient make lifestyle changes. These lifestyle changes eventually help patients improve their overall health and personal well-being.

Specific vs Overarching Goals

Most people are not able to change their behavior in one day. Lasting behavior change takes time and a lot of effort. Often, patients need help breaking down a large challenge into more manageable pieces that are easier to accomplish. You can play a crucial role in this process, by assisting the person who has one or more chronic conditions set realistic goals that he or she can achieve in a short period. We all have patients who would love to reach the stars and feel they need to set very ambitious goals. When working with such patients, our work is to help them understand the distinction between an overarching goal or outcome, on the one hand, and specific and achievable action steps over a short period, on the other.

How to Set Goals

Some patients may have a hard time identifying what they would like to work on. In these cases, you may want to help them identify something they previously tried and had success with. Is there anything that they would like to continue working on? Are there barriers they have identified that got in their way? What did they do to overcome them? Identifying barriers and having a plan in place to handle them is another important part of the goal-setting process.

The goal-setting process in the empowerment approach consists of five steps that help patients identify the information they need to develop and reach their health and lifestyle-related goals (2,5). Box 3.1 outlines these steps, along with questions you might use when working with patients (2). Note that most of these questions are open-ended. This communication technique elicits more information and provides more opportunity for dialogue than asking questions with a limited range of responses (such as "yes" or "no"). For more information on open-ended questions, refer to Chapter 5.

BOX 3.1 *Five Steps for Setting Goals*

Step I: Explore the Problem or Issue (Past)

- "What is the hardest thing about caring for your health condition?"
- "Please tell me more about that."
- "Are there some specific examples you can give me?"

Step II: Clarify Feelings and Meaning (Present)

- "What are your thoughts about this?"
- "Are you feeling (insert feeling) because (insert meaning)?"

Step III: Develop a Plan (Future)

- "What do you want?"
- "How would this situation have to change for you to feel better about it?"
- "Where would you like to be regarding this situation in (specific time, eg, 1 month, 3 months, 1 year)?"
- "What are your options?"
- "What are barriers for you?"
- "Who could help you?"
- "What are the costs and benefits for each of your choices?"

(continues)

BOX 3.1 *(continued)*

- "What would happen if you do not do anything about it?"
- "How important is it, on a scale of 1 to 10, for you to do something about this?"
- "Let's develop a plan."

Step IV: Commit to Action (Future)

- "Are you willing to do what you need to do to solve this problem?"
- "What are some steps you could take?"
- "What are you going to do?"
- "When are you going to do it?"
- "How will you know if you have succeeded?"
- "What is one thing you will do when you leave here today?"

Step V: Experience and Evaluate the Plan (Future)

- "How did it go?"
- "What did you learn?"
- "What barriers did you encounter?"
- "What, if anything, would you do differently next time?"
- "What will you do when you leave here today?"

Source: Adapted from Funnell MM, Anderson RM. Empowerment and self-management of diabetes. *Clin Diabetes.* 2004;22:123–127. Copyright 2004 American Diabetes Association. Reproduced by permission of the American Diabetes Association.

In the first two steps of the process described in Box 3.1 ("Explore the problem or issue" and "Clarify feelings and meaning"), patients have the opportunity to define the problem. They also have a chance to explore their feelings, thoughts, and beliefs that may obstruct or help with goal achievement.

The third step ("Develop a plan") is very important. As patients develop a long-term goal, they need to identify what will work and what will not. Knowing the barriers to success is critical. In addition to discussing potential barriers, you can help the patient identify experiences or support that will help with goal achievement.

In the fourth step ("Commit to action"), the patient is ready to commit to her goal. During this step, you can help the patient be very specific and realistic, so she has a clear idea of what she wants to accomplish. Imagine a patient does not currently walk as far as the mailbox. If she sets a goal of walking 45 minutes a day, 7 days a week, she is being very specific but not realistic! Your role is to guide the patient toward what will work for her. (See Chapter 6 for more information on helping patients set goals that have a high probability of success.)

The final step in empowered goal setting includes evaluation. At this point, patients state what they have learned in the process. Help your patients keep things in perspective during this last step. Some patients are not able to achieve the goals they chose and subsequently feel they have failed. How can we help patients in these circumstances?

When talking with patients in the evaluation process, consider using the term "experiments" instead of "goals." Scientists are not bad scientists because their experiment did not work. They just need to try a different approach to achieve their purpose. Similarly, if patients are not able to achieve their goals, they are not bad or failures; instead, they need to approach the challenge from a different perspective. Perhaps their goals were not realistic or lacked specificity. Perhaps they need to address other barriers or issues (3). People working on goals may be encouraged by Thomas Edison's attitude during his quest to invent the electric light: "I have not failed. I've just found 10,000 ways that won't work."

Practice Exercises

Exercise 1

As you work with patients this week, consider starting some of the sessions with open-ended questions, such as the questions listed in the first step of Box 3.1.

Exercise 2

Consider your own life and explore a concern you have by asking yourself open-ended questions. (Example: I am not making time to be physically active even though I know it is good for my physical and mental health. What is the hardest part about being active? What am I willing to do to be more active?) Write down what you would like to accomplish.

References

1. Rubin RR, Anderson RM, Funnell MM. Collaborative diabetes care. *Pract Diabetol.* 2002;21:29–32.
2. Funnell MM, Anderson RM. Empowerment and self-management of diabetes. *Clin Diabetes.* 2004;22:123–127.
3. Glasgow RE, Anderson RM. In diabetes care, moving from compliance to adherence is not enough: something entirely different is needed [letter]. *Diabetes Care.* 1999;22:2090–2092.
4. Funnell MM, Anderson RM, Arnold MS, Barr PA, Donnelly MB, Johnson PD, Taylor-Moon D, White NH. Empowerment: an idea whose time has come in diabetes education. *Diabetes Educ.* 1991;17:37–41.
5. Anderson RM, Funnell MM, Barr PA, Dedrick RF, Davis WK. Learning to empower patients. *Diabetes Care.* 1991;14:584–590.

Are Your Patients Ready to Change?

To work on a specific goal with a patient (especially a patient who was referred by another health care professional), you first determine how ready the person is to work on the goal. As we mentioned in Chapter 3, open-ended questions are a key technique in goal setting. This communication method may be tied in with two other approaches: the transtheoretical model, perhaps better known as the stages of change model, and motivational interviewing. While the transtheoretical model and motivational interviewing are two distinctive methods, they are both patient-focused and can help you identify the priorities of a patient and move the patient toward effective goal setting and accomplishment. This chapter will explore the stages of change model. See Chapter 5 for discussion of motivational interviewing.

Transtheoretical Model

Clinicians use the transtheoretical (stages of change) model to identify how ready a person is to initiate a particular behavior change. In the late 1970s and early 1980s, James Prochaska and Carlo DiClemente at the University of Rhode Island developed this model based on studies of how smokers were able to give up their habits. The idea behind their work is that behavior change does not happen in one step. Rather, most people have the tendency to progress through multiple stages on their way to a successful change. According to this model, a person can be "staged" based on his or her interest in and readiness to make a change (1). Understanding a particular patient's stage or level of change helps you determine how to approach the person regarding a specific issue.

The stages of change are as follows (2):

- **Precontemplation**—the person is not ready to make a change. He or she does not see that his or her behavior is a problem.
- **Contemplation**—the person is considering making a change but not right away. He or she knows the behavior is a problem but is not ready to make a change yet.
- **Preparation**—the person is getting ready to make a change soon.
- **Action**—the person has already taken steps toward making a change. Generally, only about 15% of people you initially meet with will be in the action stage.
- **Maintenance**—the person made a change and has been successfully working on it for at least the past 6 months.
- **Relapse**—the person has returned to the old behavior.

- **Termination**—the changed behavior has become a habit, and the person is absolutely certain that relapse will not occur.

The Significance of Staging

Remember Bob from Chapter 1? His doctor had told him that it would be a good idea to work with a registered dietitian (RD) on weight loss and learn how to eat healthfully. In their initial session, the RD followed her own agenda and made recommendations for Bob without assessing his readiness to change. The session was counterproductive. Bob did not follow her advice or return for another visit. Imagine how the outcome might have been different if the RD had used the stages of change model. She would have recognized that Bob seemed to be in the precontemplation stage. He was not ready to hear her advice and, frankly, didn't see how his behavior was problematic.

Sometimes patients may not be ready to take action on a particular goal, especially if they did not set that goal. Resist the urge to use your expertise to "fix" such patients by telling them what to do. Instead, ask open-ended questions and listen carefully to the patient's answers to find out where he is and how he feels about a particular behavior change, as well as what he wants to do. As you listen, determine where the patient fits in the stages of change model. Remember, when the patient determines what goal he is willing to set, he is typically ready to work on this behavior. You will find that letting the patient set his own goals is the best approach, as it allows both the patient and you to have a positive and productive interaction.

In this chapter, we discuss how to identify the stage a person is in, and we suggest ways to approach a patient in each stage. When you start counseling a patient, your work will focus on helping this person progress from one stage to another, until he or she reaches the action phase. Later, when patients start making progress, you will employ strategies to help prevent relapse or moving back to earlier stages and old habits. As "change agents," we need to remember change is not a straight line. In fact, people often move back and forth through various stages of readiness before they begin to take action. It's human nature!

Moving Through the Stages of Change (Jane's Story: Part 1)

Now let's meet Jane, a busy woman who is at risk for developing diabetes. Her physician referred her to an RD, Kate, for weight-loss advice and support. At Jane's first appointment, Kate starts with an open-ended question: "How important is it for you to lose weight?" Jane's answer helps Kate to "stage" her and plan an approach for going forward with Jane.

Precontemplation

The following are some signs a person is in the precontemplation stage:

- She denies having a problem.
- She makes excuses (the "yes, but" syndrome).
- She blames other people for her problems.

Jane, for example, may say she is too busy to prepare healthful food or it costs too much. She may even blame her husband for bringing the "wrong" foods into the house.

Precontemplation is the stage of resistance or reluctance, when patients may not be well informed about the benefits of a particular behavior change. You may see a need to educate them. However, to demonstrate to your patients that *they* are in charge of changing personal behavior, always ask them for permission before providing additional information.

Patients may have tried to make changes in the past but did not achieve success. They may think that a particular change is just not possible, despite knowing how important it may be. In these situations, you can help them overcome their lack of confidence regarding the issue. See Box 4.1 for additional counseling tips for the precontemplation stage.

BOX 4.1 *Counseling Tips for the Precontemplation Stage*

- Acknowledge that your patient is not ready to make changes like losing weight or changing her diet. Accept that the patient may also not view a behavior change goal as important right now.
- Affirm that the decision of what to do or not to do is entirely up to the patient.
- Encourage the patient to consider the positive aspects of making a change.
- Discuss what the patient thinks he or she *is* willing to change.

After they talk, Kate understands that Jane may not be ready to make any diet changes right now, even though she came to the session to learn about healthful eating. Jane may have initially focused on "diet changes" because her conversation with her physician led her to believe that eating is what she needs to change. Healthful eating may not really be her personal concern, or it may be an area that she has a low level of confidence in addressing.

However, she states that she is willing to start taking walks in the evening.

Remember that a patient in the precontemplation stage in one area may be ready to make a change in another area, or even within different components of an area. For example, a patient who generally skips breakfast may be ready to start eating breakfast. However, expanding the goal to include carb counting or limiting fats at breakfast may be too overwhelming at the moment. Your job is to help the patient figure out (in great detail) exactly what she is ready to do and what barriers she thinks may get in the way.

What generally *doesn't* work for people in the precontemplation stage (or at any stage for that matter) are threats of negative consequences. If you tell a person, "You are probably going to have a heart attack or stroke if you don't change your ways," she will usually ignore your statement. In fact, such threats often cause a person to "dig her heels in" and find more excuses *not* to change. If you are using threats with your patients, our advice to you is stop now! Threats just don't work!

Contemplation

Jane may recognize that her weight is a problem and may even want to do something about it. However, she has many hurdles she needs to overcome before she will be able to implement a change. She just needs to finish this big project at work, and then she can make a plan and start working on it. Or, she just has to get through the holidays—everyone expects her to bake all of the holiday treats, and the kids and grandkids will be coming for an extended visit. A person in the contemplation stage generally isn't prepared to take action for at least another 6 months. See Box 4.2 for counseling tips for the contemplation stage.

BOX 4.2 *Counseling Tips for the Contemplation Stage*

People in the contemplation stage are fence sitters. We want to help them jump off the fence and start working on behavior changes that are meaningful to them. Some techniques you can employ are the same as those you would use for the person in the precontemplation stage:

- Acknowledge that the patient may not be ready to make changes in a particular behavior (or does not view that outcome as important right now).
- Affirm that the decision of what to do or not to do is entirely up to the patient.
- Encourage the patient to consider positive aspects of making behavior changes.
- Work on the patient's ambivalence about consequences of behavior change.

Patients in the contemplation stage are often ambivalent about the consequences of behavior change, and they may need to work through that phase before they are ready to change. You may want to ask patients in this stage to consider the negative and positive consequences of *not* changing, as well as the negative and positive consequences of making the change. (We will discuss ambivalence in greater detail in Chapter 5.)

Jane undertakes this exercise and identifies some of the benefits and consequences of making food changes to help with weight loss (see Table 4.1). Once Jane has completed her list, she and Kate can discuss the pros and cons. While discussing Jane's ambivalence, Kate begins to gain fresh insight into Jane's thoughts and feelings. More importantly, Kate helps Jane reflect on what

TABLE 4.1 *Jane Considers Making a Behavior Change*

Behavior	Advantages (Pros)	Disadvantages (Cons)
Not making diet changes	Can still eat all the foods I love. Don't have to plan meals. Can still eat fast food. No one tells me what to do.	May gain more weight. May end up developing diabetes like my sister.
Making diet changes	Will lose weight, feel better, fit into clothes I have outgrown. Will feel less embarrassed about body size, be healthier.	Have to deprive myself. Will be hungry all the time, and can't eat foods I love. Need to find a different way to deal with stress.

these changes will or will not bring into her life. Jane now has a chance to evaluate what is more important for her. This conversation may help her tip the balance toward making a change. She may now be willing to discuss in more depth other things she can do to improve her health and which consequences matter to her.

Remember, if you are going to provide information to a patient, always ask her for permission first. The patient needs to be ready to hear the information.

Preparation

If Jane feels that weight loss is important and states she is ready to take action, she is probably in the preparation stage. In fact, she may have already started implementing some changes. At this stage, Kate focuses on helping Jane set an appropriate plan so she can succeed.

The patient in this stage will benefit from working on short-term goals and developing a plan for accomplishing them. Help your patients identify a measurable goal that is achievable within the next 1 to 2 weeks. You also want to help identify the barriers that could get in the way. See Box 4.3 for additional counseling tips for the preparation stage. By using these tips, you can develop a partnership with your patient. Keep in mind that the patient must be in complete control. You may have lots of great advice to offer; but the bottom line is that success depends on what the person does when she leaves your office. Your approach should focus on the person and take into account her readiness to make behavior changes.

BOX 4.3 *Counseling Tips for the Preparation Stage*

- Help patients identify who they can turn to for support, such as a spouse, friend or an actual support group.
- Reinforce that patients have the skills to achieve their goals.
- Affirm that small steps taken on a consistent basis result in success.

Action

By the action stage, you and your patients have built a successful partnership. They have set their goals and are achieving them. In this stage, you will help patients make adjustments so they can stay on track. What types of situations may make it difficult for individual patients to stick with their plans and reach their personal goals?

Jane has begun to include five to seven servings of fruit and vegetables in her diet each day. However, she is planning a vacation and will be eating out frequently. She is concerned it may be difficult to stick with her new eating habits and asks Kate for some assistance. Kate begins the discussion by asking her, "How are you planning to handle your meals while you are on vacation?" As Jane responds, Kate helps her identify possible solutions. Kate does *not* use her expertise as an RD to create a list for Jane. After Jane has made her own list, Kate asks for permission to offer some additional tips. They also role-play some scenarios to help Jane prepare for vacation eating. Kate affirms the changes Jane has made thus far, and reminds her that she has the skills to manage difficult situations.

People in the action phase are more successful if they have supportive relationships, especially at times when they are experiencing high levels of stress. Be sure to ask patients about their support systems. In addition, help them come up with healthful ways to handle temptations. For example, if nighttime snacking is a problem for Jane, taking a walk or phoning a friend may be healthful and helpful alternatives.

Maintenance

A patient in the maintenance stage has successfully adopted positive behavior changes and sustained those changes for at least 6 months. At this stage, follow-up is still important to prevent relapse. Your patients may even want to "plan for relapse" (ie, identify potential problem situations and put a plan in place). For example, Jane may be worried about the holiday meal at Thanksgiving. To plan for this potentially stressful time, she sets up appointments with Kate before and during the holidays. Kate also works with Jane to set up a Thanksgiving-specific plan to include more activity, eat healthful foods, and manage stress in positive ways. As you work with patients, ask them when they feel they may be most likely to relapse and plan strategies or visits around those situations.

During the maintenance stage, continue to help patients focus on the benefits of change. For example, Kate reminds Jane that she wants to make the meal plan change to help with weight loss so that she will feel better, prevent diabetes, and fit into her clothes.

Relapse (or Recycling)

Jane has been doing well making and sticking to behavior changes. In fact, she has lost weight and kept most of it off for over 2 years now. Her blood glucose, lipids, and blood pressure are under good control. She has not seen Kate in over 6 months. Life is good!

Kate worked with Jane in the maintenance phase to identify and plan for "trigger events." However, unexpected events like a death of a family member or friend, divorce, or job loss may lead Jane to deviate from her health plan. Even those patients who have incorporated a change into their lives for an extended period may go off track. For others, the change now seems to be second nature.

Patients may have feelings of disappointment, frustration, and failure if they relapse after having changes in place for a period of time, and they may not seek assistance. Affirm with patients that most people need more than one attempt to make a change and life circumstances may cause them to get off track in the future.

Help your patients identify a course of action to take in case they unexpectedly relapse. The action plan may include increasing the frequency of visits with you or other health care providers.

Termination

When someone reaches the termination stage, the change has become second nature. Patients in this stage are not tempted to go back to the old behavior.

A person may reach the termination phase after being in the action stage for 6 months to 5 years. Generally, the new behavior has become a habit, like buckling up the seat belt when getting in the car or brushing teeth.

However, keep in mind that for some people, certain behaviors may never reach the termination stage. For example, Jane may always have to be aware of triggers that may cause a relapse. To help her, Kate encourages her to return once or twice a year for support and to continue working on the change.

Practice Exercises

Exercise 1

If you are meeting with patients who have goals "assigned" to them by their physician, ask them how ready they are to work on the goal. Identify their stage based on their response and use the strategies outlined in the chapter.

Exercise 2

Take a look at the accomplishment or change you wanted to achieve that you wrote down in Chapter 3. Now ask yourself how motivated you are to make that change. Identify what stage you are in currently. If you are not in the action phase, write down the benefits of making a change. Use Table 4.1 as an example.

References

1. Prochaska JO, DiClemente CC, Norcross JC. In search of how people change: applications to addictive behaviors. *Am Psychol.* 1992;47:1102–1114.
2. Prochaska JO. Decision making in the transtheoretical model of behavior change. *Med Decis Making.* 2008;28:845.

5

Moving Your Patients Toward Change: Motivational Interviewing

In Chapter 4, we reviewed the stages of change model and offered some suggestions for identifying how ready a person is to make a specific behavior change. This chapter focuses on another common technique used by practitioners: motivational interviewing (MI). This approach can help patients overcome ambivalence and move toward change. Please note that to effectively use MI, training with ongoing coaching is recommended (1).

The Origins of Motivational Interviewing

The clinical psychologist William R. Miller first described MI in 1983, and at that time the technique was mainly used to treat people who had a problem with alcohol (2). He described motivation as being an interpersonal process that focuses on individual responsibility and internal desire to change. Later, Miller and

Rollnick defined motivational interviewing as a "directive, client centered counseling style for eliciting behavior change by helping clients explore and resolve ambivalence" (3). MI is a communication method that can be effective when working with patients who are struggling to change or who are ambivalent about changing their behavior. MI strategies focus on guiding patients toward change, but not on telling them what to do or attempting to "motivate" them. The practitioner is supportive of the choices the patients make, instead of telling them what is wrong with their choices, and practitioners also appeal to the internal motivation that all of us naturally have (4).

Efficacy of Motivational Interviewing

The American Dietetic Association Evidence Analysis Library examined four nutrition intervention studies that used dietitians who were trained in motivational interviewing. In all four studies, patients in the groups where MI was used achieved significantly better outcomes than the groups of patients where this strategy was not used. The improved outcomes included weight loss, better blood glucose control in people with diabetes, less consumption of fat, and adoption of low-fat methods to cook vegetables (5–8). A literature review by Cummings and colleagues showed that MI is particularly useful with older adults (9). It helped older adults with a variety of health issues that included becoming more physically active, improving their diets, lowering cholesterol and blood pressure, and improving blood glucose control. Based on these studies, the bottom line is that when MI is used with the appropriate patients by well-trained professionals who are skilled in MI, it works!

MI can help people overcome barriers to and build a personal case for change. Although motivational interviewing was initially used for treating addiction, it also can be used in the management of diseases that are directly or indirectly affected by the behavior of the person.

Basic Principles of Motivational Interviewing

Overview

MI involves several steps, along with the development of specific skills. It is a patient-centered method, in which the registered dietitian (RD) or other counselor functions more as a guide than as a teacher. The purpose is to focus on one behavior, which is selected from a menu of choices generated by the patient, at a time (10). When you use this technique, you ask strategic questions and then listen carefully to the patient's responses so you can determine whether the patient is willing to and interested in making a particular lifestyle change. If a person is not yet ready to make changes, "pushing" for a change can be counterproductive. Trying to make a patient institute a change before he or she is ready is like trying to get a 2-year-old to swallow a medication that tastes bad—the harder you try, the more the child resists. Most of us have some of that willful child in us—someone telling us what we should do can make us dig in our heels and do just the opposite.

With MI, you can help the patient explore why he or she is resistant to or ambivalent about making a change. For example, why does a patient express frustration about not losing weight while continuing to make choices that are not consistent with this goal? Using questions, reflections, and other strategies consistent with MI, you can guide the patient through what is holding him back from or getting in the way of a self-selected change. Throughout the process, the patient decides whether she wants to make a change and what she wants to change, and then she sets her own goal. You are an adviser, asking questions to help the person identify an area of concern and develop a plan that she wants to and is confident she can accomplish. You may also offer suggestions, after first asking the patient if she is open to hearing your ideas. The most important things to remember are to listen more, advise less, and ask open-ended questions.

Table 5.1 (11) provides an overview of what MI is and is not. As we shall explore in the pages to follow, motivational interviewing helps patients identify *ambivalence,* which is a necessary first step toward moving them into action and changing behavior. *Empathy* is a key part of this collaborative approach; you will want to exhibit a willingness to understand the thoughts and feelings of your patients. As part of this, you will need to be comfortable with open-ended questions, affirmations, reflective listening, and summaries, while providing the patients with a safe and accepting environment that helps them express their personal thoughts, feelings, and experiences. As we have mentioned, the patients determine the pace and the direction of counseling. It is critical for patients to be in control if you want them to be invested in changing their behaviors. In addition, you'll want to avoid overloading the conversation with advice and direct teaching (2,10).

Ambivalence

Addressing ambivalence (ie, being unsure of what direction to follow) is the cornerstone of motivational interviewing. A person who experiences ambivalence will often perceive advantages and disadvantages in both maintaining a current behavior and changing to a new behavior. When you are working on ambivalence with a patient, you may want to use the technique we discussed in "Contemplation" section of Jane's story in Chapter 4—ask the patient to consider the negative and positive consequences of *not* changing as well as the negative and positive consequences of making the

TABLE 5.1 *What Is Motivational Interviewing (MI)?*

MI Is . . .	MI Is *Not* . . .
Patient-directed	A health care provider leading the discussion and making decisions for the patient
A partnership between the patient and the health care provider	Trying to persuade a patient to change
Accepting of where the patient is	Confrontational regarding patient behavior
A health care provider primarily asking the patient questions to help her resolve ambivalence to change	Focused on the health care provider giving advice to the patient
Viewing resistance to change as normal	Using "noncompliant" to label patients

Source: Data are from reference 11: Rollnick S, Miller WR. What is motivational interviewing? http://www.motivationalinterview.org/clinical/whatismi.html. Accessed March 5, 2011.

change. This way, the patient has a chance of seeing the pros and cons of making a change or not making a change. With the patient, you can also spend some time looking at perceived barriers to change and guide her toward naming solutions to barriers (12).

Table 5.2 (page 58) is an example of a decisional balance tool that you may use to help someone having difficulty committing to a course of action to explore advantages and disadvantages of change vs status quo. (We have already seen how this tool can be used in the case study of Jane in Table 4.1 of Chapter 4.) While decisional balance tools may be helpful, they are not an integral part of MI. They may allow some patients to more clearly see what

TABLE 5.2 *Decisional Balance Tool for Exploring Ambivalence*

Behavior	Advantages (Pros)	Disadvantages (Cons)
Not making the behavior change	What do you like about your current behaviors?	What don't you like about staying the same?
Making the behavior change	What good will happen as a result of making a change?	What don't you like about making a change?

is influencing their decisions regarding change, but they are not necessary for every patient (10).

Motivational interviewing regards ambivalence as a part of the natural process of altering one's behavior, a phase that people have to go through before they can change. As we have noted in previous chapters, some RDs feel that they need to lecture patients about the benefits of eating healthier food. These RDs understandably want to share their wealth of knowledge. However, this approach often results in the patient becoming even more resistant to change. While the RD is trying to "push" the patient into adopting a new behavior, the patient is selling himself on why he doesn't want to change (12). For example, imagine a patient who is debating whether to avoid eating a bedtime snack two times a week.

Open-Ended Questions

We mentioned in Chapters 3 and 4 the importance of using open-ended questions to elicit discussions with your patients. In this section, we will explore in more detail how you can implement these questions when using MI techniques. Open-ended questions are a great conversation-starting tool to use in social settings, too! Here are some examples (12):

- **Tell me more.** Example: "Tell me how you feel about having this condition."
- **What?** Examples: "What is the most difficult thing about changing your eating habits?" "What is the hardest thing about having diabetes?"
- **How?** Example: "How do you feel when your blood glucose is over 200 most of the time?"

Think twice before using the word "why" to begin an open-ended question, especially if the question could sound judgmental. "Why?" can cause people to think you are blaming or scolding them, as in "Why did you eat so many snacks this week?" On the other hand, a well-phrased "why" question could help you and your patient understand better what is happening. An example is, "Why do you think it is so difficult to make time to walk after work?"

Avoid closed-ended questions like, "Did you take your insulin as directed this week?" This type of question puts the patient in a passive role where only a simple "yes" or "no" is required, and then the ball is back in your court. Ask instead, "How did you use your insulin this week?"

Affirmations

Each time you meet with a patient, find something—large or small—to affirm about him. Such affirmations can help you to build a positive relationship with your patient. In addition, affirmations can help increase a patient's self-efficacy.

An affirmation and praise are not the same. The big difference is that in an affirmation you communicate the "value" of the person and her behavior, while praise may be perceived as passing judgment on behavior. An example of an affirmation is, "Following your action plan helped you lose 10 pounds over the past 4 months." In contrast, an example of praise is, "Congratulations, I am so proud of you for losing 10 pounds" (12).

Reflective Listening

The reflective listening technique is an integral skill to develop when using the MI approach. To use this technique, listen carefully and then repeat or restate what the patient just told you. Pose your response as a statement, not a question. By repeating back what the patient said, you give the patient the opportunity to affirm that you understand or to clarify because your interpretation is incorrect (12).

Reflective listening thus shows a patient you are listening and you understand what they are saying. The effective use of reflective listening also keeps the conversation moving forward, closer to goal setting and behavior change (13). Just be careful not to overuse this approach. You do not want to sound like you are repeating every single thing your patient is saying. The following is an example of a script you might use:

> **Patient:** "It's just too hard. I don't want to change my diet."
> **RD:** "You don't want to change your diet because you find it easier to keep it the same."

Alternately, you may rephrase what the patient just said:

> **Patient:** "I really want to start exercising again."
> **RD:** "Sounds like you are ready to start exercising again."

You may want to reframe what the patient said to put a positive and encouraging spin on it:

Patient: "I have tried so many times to lose weight, but I am never successful."

RD: "Your efforts say a lot about your perseverance and how important weight control is for you. Even though it has been difficult for you, you don't give up!"

Rolling with Resistance

Directly challenging a patient about their lifestyle behavior is counterproductive because the confrontation typically results in the patient defending his current behavior. Instead, MI advocates the principle of "rolling with resistance." When you roll with resistance, you give recognition to the normal ambivalence that is part of being human. From this perspective, resistance is viewed as a normal process to be expected, rather than as a threat to your authority or expertise. So, instead of meeting a patient's resistance head on, you acknowledge the resistance and step aside, figuratively speaking. When you acknowledge resistance, it tends to lose its intensity. If you align with the patient to address the issues together, the energy behind the resistance can sometimes be channeled into small steps toward change. However, this is not to imply that you can never disagree with a patient's viewpoint (14).

Summaries

Summaries are a nice way to move from one topic to the next, or to highlight some of the ambivalence that you have identified in the patient. You may also want to use a summary at the end of the appointment to recap the major points of discussion (11). When you summarize, you generally start with a statement that describes what you and your patient talked about. After making this statement, you then list some of the key items you and your patient have just discussed. This is a point where you can also refer to any ambivalence that you and the patient noted. You then invite the patient to add anything to the summary that you may have missed. To end a summary while keeping the conversation moving forward, ask an open-ended question (13).

Providing Advice

With MI, you reserve your advice for the patient until late in the conversation. This last phase comes into play after the patient states what she wants to do. If you have concerns about her thinking on the subject, ask for permission to share some thoughts with her. If she grants permission, you can then offer suggestions and share some of what you learned from those years of education and experience! But be careful—remember the patient's opinion is what matters most, not yours.

What to Do When a Patient Clams Up or Spouts Off

Sometimes it may seem like you just are not connecting with a patient. He may be quick to argue, ignore you, or answer "Yes, but." When this happens, remember that communication is a two-way street. If you are feeling frustrated about your conversation with a patient, he is likely feeling the same way. Your conversation may be entering an area the patient is not ready to explore, or you may be giving advice when he is not ready to receive it.

The following are few things to ask yourself in these situations:

- Do I really know how the patient feels about this topic? Ask the patient if he is interested in or ready to address the issue. The transtheoretical (stages of change) model we discussed in Chapter 4 may help you "stage" the person.
- Why is the patient feeling so strongly about this?
- Am I allowing the patient to control which issues we discuss or am I preempting her?
- Am I being a teacher and telling the patient what to do?
- Have I been listening more than talking?

Next, take steps to diffuse the situation (12):

- Make sure you are using reflective listening.
- Empathize with the patient and normalize actions—"Most people make several attempts before they are able to lose weight."
- Disclose something about your own experiences, if appropriate. "I also used to be overweight. Even as a dietitian with all the right knowledge, I had a difficult time making diet and physical activity changes." Keep any self-disclosure short and simple. The appointment is about your patient, not you.
- Get back to asking what the patient wants to talk about.
- Make certain the patient knows your goal is not to "make" him change. You are simply there to support what the person wants, which may or may not include behavior change.

Optimizing the Results of Motivational Interviewing

When coupled with other interventions, MI can be an even more powerful tool in patient behavior change. What else do we need to do to help our patients? Based on a systematic literature review and meta-analysis, Rubak and colleagues (4) concluded that the time spent with the patient, the frequency of the visits, and the length of the visits were equally important in helping a patient make changes. The following are some of the points to take away from this research:

- Meet with each patient several times, if possible. When MI was used in one encounter with patients, about 40% of them showed a positive effect. When the number of encounters was five or more, the number of patients making changes increased to 87%!
- Longer sessions may be more successful than shorter sessions, but brief encounters (eg, 15 minutes) are still useful—81% of subjects in sessions that were 60 minutes in length showed positive changes, and 64% showed a positive effect when sessions were briefer than 20 minutes.
- Follow-up is key. Among participants who were followed for at least 1 year, 81% showed improvement, whereas 36% showed positive effects when followed for 3 months.
- The impact of MI is closely related to the duration and number of encounters between the patient and the provider and less strongly associated with the education the patient received. Practitioners trained in MI make a difference in patient outcomes!
- Practice your listening skills with patients and/or family members. If you want a real challenge, try it out with a teenager who has been giving you grief!

Jeff's Story: Part 2

Remember Jeff from Chapter 3? He was the busy CEO who found it difficult to follow the RD's advice regarding weight control and diabetes self-management. Here's an example of how a follow-up visit might go if the RD (whom we'll call Kris) used traditional communication techniques:

> **Kris:** Jeff, I see that you have gained weight and that your blood glucose is up—a lot.
>
> **Jeff:** I know. I just do not have time to make all those changes.
>
> **Kris:** Would you rather have a heart attack or stroke, or lose your eyesight?
>
> **Jeff:** No.
>
> **Kris:** Well if you don't make some changes, you can be sure to wreck your health!!
>
> **Jeff:** It is not that bad. I know several people with diabetes who are doing just fine. The doctor increased my medication; I think that is all I need.
>
> **Kris:** Watching what you eat and exercising are also important.
>
> **Jeff:** That may be true, but what if I do not have time for that?
>
> **Kris:** Do you have time to be dead or disabled?
>
> **Jeff:** Just give me another meal plan, and I will see if I can follow it. But I am not going to exercise; I am too tired for that.

Kris and Jeff begin talking about some meal planning ideas, but how committed do you think Jeff is to this plan? Did Kris listen, or was she stuck on giving advice (and making threats)? Now let's replay the encounter with Kris using MI techniques:

> **Kris:** Jeff, tell me, what your biggest concern is today? *(Start with an open-ended question.)*

Jeff: I am too busy to make time for physical activity and to change my diet. But I am concerned about gaining more weight and my blood pressure and sugar levels being so high. Also, I am tired all the time!

Kris: It sounds like you are concerned about your health and making time for being more active and eating differently are difficult for you to fit in. In addition, you are tired. *(Note: Kris is using reflective listening.)*

Jeff: That's right—I just don't know what to do! This health change stuff on top of work is too much for me to deal with right now. And I don't have the energy for it!

Kris: Making many changes when you are busy and feeling more tired is overwhelming.

Jeff: Yeah, that's right! What am I supposed to do?? *(Note: In some circumstances, it may be helpful to screen patients like Jeff for depression; for more details, see Chapter 7.)*

Kris: I think I hear you say that you cannot handle making several lifestyle changes now. Can you name one thing that you think you would be able to address?

Jeff: Well, I have to eat, and I eat out all the time. I think I need more help with choosing different options when I eat out. Will that help my energy level too?

Kris: Eating out sounds like a great starting point. What do you know about diabetes, food, and your energy level?

Jeff: I know food makes the sugar go up and exercise can help it come down. In addition, the doctor gave me this medication, metformin, that is supposed to help my blood sugar. He just increased the dose, too. And high blood sugar can make you feel tired! *(Note: Instead of "lecturing" or "educating," Kris allows Jeff to tell her what he knows.)*

Kris: So, making different food choices and looking at the amount of food you eat can help keep your blood sugar from going up too much, and the medication will help too! And keeping blood sugar from going too high can help you feel less tired.

At this point Kris can now spend some time exploring with Jeff how he eats and the types of foods and drinks he chooses when eating out. She can then ask him what he thinks would be reasonable to change. While exploring with Jeff what he thinks he could do differently, Kris may find opportunities to ask for permission to offer some education on food choices. Her next step will be to help guide Jeff through the goal-setting process, which we will discuss in greater detail in Chapter 6.

Practice Exercises

Exercise 1

Be on the lookout for patient resistance. If you detect it, ask yourself the question, "Am I addressing the patient's concerns?" Also, check to see whether you are listening more than talking. Are you asking open-ended questions? Do you need to limit your advice giving and lecturing?

Exercise 2

Practice reflective listening with patients using techniques listed in this chapter—repeating, paraphrasing, or offering a positive spin.

Exercise 3

Consider asking one or two patients if you can tape your sessions to help you improve how you work with others.

References

1. Miller WR, Rollnick S. Ten things that motivational interviewing is not. *Behav Cognit Psychol*. 2009;37:129–140.
2. Miller WR. Motivational interviewing with problem drinkers. *Behav Psychother*. 1983;11:147–172.
3. Miller WR, Rollnick S. *Motivational Interviewing: Preparing People to Change Addictive Behavior*. New York, NY: Guildford Press; 2002.
4. Rubak S, Sandbaek A, Lauritzen T, Christensen B. Motivational interviewing: a systematic review and meta-analysis. *Br J Gen Pract*. 2005;55:305–312.

5. Bowen D, Ehret C, Pedersen M, Snetselaar L, Johnson M, Tinker L, Hollinger D, Lichty I, Bland K, Sivertsen D, Ocken D, Staats L, Beedoe JW. Results of an adjunct dietary intervention program in the Women's Health Initiative. *J Am Diet Assoc.* 2002;102:1631–1637.

6. Resnicow K, Jackson A, Wang T, De AK, McCarty F, Dudley WN, Baranowski T. A motivational interviewing intervention to increase fruit and vegetable intake through black churches: results of the Eat for Life Trial. *Am J Public Health.* 2001;91:1686–1692.

7. Smith DE, Heckemeyer CM, Kratt PP, Mason DA. Motivational interviewing to improve adherence to behavioral weight control program for older obese women with NIDDM. *Diabetes Care.* 1997;20:52–54.

8. West DS, DiLillo V, Bursac Z, Gore SA, Greene PG. Motivational interviewing improves weight loss in women with type 2 diabetes. *Diabetes Care.* 2007;30:1081–1087.

9. Cummings SM. Motivational interviewing to affect behavioral change in older adults. *Res Social Work Pract.* 2005;19:195–204.

10. American Association of Diabetes Educators. *The Art and Science of Self-Management Education: A Desk Reference for Health Care Professionals.* Chicago, IL: American Association of Diabetes Educators; 2006.

11. Rollnick S, Miller WR. What is motivational interviewing? http://www.motivationalinterview.org/clinical/whatismi.html. Accessed March 5, 2011.

12. Borrelli B. Using motivational interviewing to promote patient behavior change and enhance health. http://www/medscape.com/viewprogram/5757_pnt. Accessed June 1, 2009.

13. Wagner C, Conners W. Motivational interviewing: interaction techniques. http://motivationalinterview.org/clinical/interaction.html. Accessed September 9, 2010.

14. VanWormer JJ, Boucher JL. Motivational interviewing and diet modification: a review of the evidence. *Diabetes Educ.* 2004;30:404–414.

6

Putting the *WHAT* into Goal Setting

"The reason most people never reach their goals is that they don't define them, or ever seriously consider them as believable or achievable. Winners can tell you where they are going, what they plan to do along the way, and who will be sharing the adventure with them."

—DENIS WAITLEY

Most of our patients have heard advice from their health care professionals like lose weight, exercise more, cut down on saturated fat, reduce your salt intake, or get more fiber into your diet. Unfortunately, many of our patients do not know how to translate these broad goals into their everyday lives. As registered dietitians (RDs), we can help our patients quantify and develop action plans around outcomes like "eat less saturated fat" or "lose weight."

In previous chapters, we talked about letting patients set their own agendas—each patient should determine what she is interested in working on. Your next objective is to guide patients into action. Once they are ready to make a change and have identified where they would like to start, you will help them set achievable goals. One key to setting goals is *desire*—the goal has to be something the patient wants to do. The second key is *confidence*—the goal needs to be something the patient is fairly certain she can accomplish. The third key, which we will cover in this chapter, is how to help your patients set *very specific goals* or action plans. Finally, to succeed in achieving their goals, patients also need frequent follow-up (1–4).

Fostering Confidence

If patients have desire and confidence, they should be able to successfully initiate health changes, with your guidance and support. Self-efficacy (or confidence) is one's ability to change and achieve healthier behaviors. Bodenheimer and colleagues showed that even patients who have a low income level and obtain their care through safety-net clinics were able to set and achieve goals as often as higher income patients who were seen in private practices, as long as they wanted to change and believed it was possible for them to change (5).

In Chapter 7, we will go into more detail about emotional health issues and other stressors that may prevent a person from having the desire and confidence to change. These obstacles can include high anxiety levels, depression, a lack of money, family concerns, or competing time issues. For some patients, the first steps may be to identify any such concerns in their lives and to find out where to go for assistance. Until they take these steps, they cannot embark on lifestyle changes such as increasing physical activity, healthier eating, or tobacco cessation.

As we mentioned in Chapter 3, some patients may feel more confident if they view the goal as an experiment. This way, if they do not achieve it, they may be less likely to perceive themselves as failures.

The WHAT System

As we have discussed in previous chapters, patients who are ready to change will be more successful if they set their own goals. Broad objectives are not enough. Goals must be specific and achievable, tailored to the individual's lifestyle and culture. To help your patients with goal setting, we created the **WHAT** system:

- **W** stands for *what* will the patient do, *when* will he or she do it, and *where* will he or she do it.
- **H** is for *how much* or *how many*, and *how often*.
- **A** stands for *achievable* (and believable).
- **T** represents the *time frame* for accomplishing the goal.

The more precise the goal or action plan is, the easier it will be for the patient to incorporate it into his or her life. See Table 6.1 (page 74) for tips on refining initial goals so they are specific and achievable.

Jane's Story: Part 2

You met Jane and her RD, Kate, in Chapter 4. Jane is interested in losing weight and is willing to make some diet changes to achieve that objective. How can Kate use WHAT to help her?

What, When, and Where?

Let's start with **W**—*what* will the patient do, *when* will she do it, and *where* will she do it? To start with goal setting, Kate asks for permission to advise Jane on potential meal plan changes that may help with weight loss. Jane settles on incorporating more fruits and vegetables in her eating plan—that action is the *what*.

TABLE 6.1 *Goal-Setting Tips*

Original Goal	Concerns	Techniques to Improve Goal	Possible New Action Step
Lose weight.	Action is not specific.	Identify action linked with weight loss that patient wants to try.	I will walk 20 minutes after dinner on M, W, and F.
Walk more, eat less, drink more water, avoid sweets, eat more vegetables, lift weights, do yoga.	Too many goals.	Help patient choose one or two specific goals to work on and track.	Pack fresh veggies as part of lunch M-F this week. Have salad with dinner M, W, and F this week.
My doctor said I should avoid white flour and sugar.	Goal does not identify what patient wants to do.	Help patient set reasonable action plan. Communicate with doctor. of patient	I will drink water or diet soda in place of regular soda once per day (M to F). I will buy whole grain bread to use in place of white bread for sandwiches.
Eat less.	Goal is too vague.	Help patient create a specific action plan.	I will drink only water after dinner (no snacks or calorie-containing liquids) 5 days this week (Sun thru Thurs).

Then Kate asks Jane *when* she wants to work on incorporating more fruits and vegetables. Jane decides to start with lunch—she often brings a lunch from home to work and frequently supplements it with vending machine items like chips and candy. She decides that she will bring some fruit and veggies to work as part of her lunch instead of purchasing items from the vending machine. In making this plan, Jane also answers *where*—she will work on her goal at her worksite.

How?

Now the questions to ask are *how much* or *how many,* and *how often.* Jane decides that she will supplement her lunch with one piece of fruit and a small bag of raw veggies (thus answering, "How many?"). For *how often,* Jane says that she wants to do this every workday—that is, Monday through Friday.

Achievability

Next Kate helps Jane determine whether this goal is *achievable* for her. Does Jane *believe* that she will be able to pack fruit and raw vegetables for every lunch and not use the vending machines? To make it easier for her to avoid vending machine purchases, Jane said she will leave her cash at home. There is no ATM nearby, and she usually uses her credit or debit cards for other types of purchases. Plus, she knows that she would not feel comfortable asking her coworkers to loan her money for vending machine purchases. Jane also decides to stock up on different kinds of fruits and vegetables when she does her weekly shopping.

Time Frame

Now for the *time frame*. Typically, you will help patients set an action plan or goal that can be accomplished during the next 1 to 2 weeks and then have them follow-up with you at the end of the time period. Sometimes people find they have problems achieving their goals, despite your best efforts to help them develop a WHAT plan. If that is the case, you will want to help the person revise his plan sooner instead of later. If the goal does not work, some people will throw up their hands and give up on the goal. If they know they are going to check in with someone regarding their goals, they are often less likely to totally dismiss their action plan. Understanding this, Kate sets up a follow-up visit for Jane in 2 weeks.

Putting WHAT into Action

Before the action plan is launched, Kate can verbally summarize the goal for Jane—to bring a piece of fruit and a bag of veggies for lunch from Monday through Friday for the next 2 weeks—and invite her to write it down, if she desires. If Jane seems hesitant to write out her goal, Kate could also offer to write it down for Jane. However, it can be empowering to patients if they write it out themselves. Once the goal is written, Kate shares with Jane that some people find it helpful to post the goal in a visible location and track their progress through keeping a log.

Next Kate takes the final step in setting the goal—she affirms Jane's confidence level in achieving her action plan. Kate asks Jane to use a 0-to-10 confidence scale to measure her certainty of whether or not she can accomplish her action plan (Figure 6.1). Zero means that she is absolutely sure she *cannot* meet her goal and 10 indicates that she is completely certain that she *will* do it.

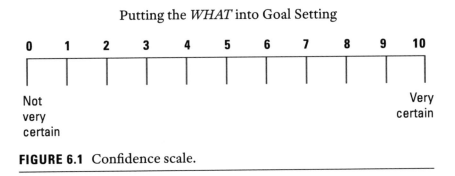

FIGURE 6.1 Confidence scale.

People who score 7 or higher on the confidence scale are most likely to succeed. If Jane does not score at least 7, Kate will want to help her adjust her goal. Jane says the goal will be a big change for her; but she wants to make the change and she is fairly certain that she will be successful. She rates her confidence level as a 7.

Following Up: Adjusting the Goal as Needed

At her follow-up visit, Jane shares her progress toward achieving her goal with Kate. Jane reports that she was not completely successful. The first week she brought the fruit and veggies every day, but she ate them on only 4 out of 5 days. On the fifth day, she went out to lunch. The following week, she brought and ate the fruit and vegetables on 3 days, and she did not have time to prepare veggies for the fourth and fifth days. On those days, she brought money to work to purchase items from the vending machine.

Jane's account illustrates why follow-up is so critical. Jane was successful some of the time. The follow-up appointment is an opportunity for Kate to remind Jane that this is an experiment and to help her problem-solve or redefine her goal. Kate asks, "What got in the way of you achieving your action plan?" Jane replies that she likes to eat out with her friends at lunch a couple of times a month. Kate then asks Jane if she would like to revise her goal so that she can accommodate eating out at lunch. Jane says perhaps 4 days a week of bringing the fruit and veggies for lunch would be more realistic. Kate also asks about Jane "not having time" to prepare vegetables. "Is there something that you would do differently so that you make certain you have veggies ready and available for lunch?"

In situations like Jane's, you may find that patients don't seem to have a ready solution in mind. To help Jane problem-solve, Kate uses a technique known as "brainstorming." The brainstorming guidelines listed in Box 6.1 are based on those used in the Stanford Chronic Disease Self-Management Program (6).

BOX 6.1 *Brainstorming Guidelines to Use When Following Up with Patients*

1. Patient identifies a problem (write the problem down for the patient to see).
2. Ask the patient to list possible solutions.
3. Request that the patient not analyze the solutions during the brainstorming.
4. The patient should just throw out ideas that come to mind—no idea is stupid. Promote creativity when the patient is listing ideas.
5. Write the ideas down for the patient.
6. If you have additional ideas, ask the patient if you can add a couple of ideas to the list.
7. Ask the patient if she would like to try one of the ideas on the list.

In response to Jane's comment that she ran out of time to pre-pare vegetables, Kate asks her if she would like to think of ways to make sure she has veggies ready for her lunch. Jane lists some ideas, such as shop more often, buy vegetables that are already cut up, or leave a big bag in the office refrigerator so she doesn't have to prepare them every day. Kate asks for permission to add other ideas to her list, and then suggests that Jane buy frozen or canned vegetables, keep some frozen or canned vegetables at work, make casseroles that have extra vegetables in them to take to work, or consider purchasing some dried vegetables.

Next Kate asks Jane to consider what is on the list and identify one possible solution she would like to try over the next week. Jane looks the list over and states she hadn't really thought about keeping frozen vegetables at work. She feels she would like to in-corporate that into her action plan.

Kate asks Jane to define her revised goal. Kate listens care-fully, in case Jane needs some WHAT guidance. Once again, Kate asks Jane about her confidence level. Kate wants to make certain that Jane leaves with a well-defined goal she feels confident that she can accomplish.

Kate then arranges for a follow-up appointment with Jane. She also reaffirms the successes Jane had over the past 2 weeks and reinforces the reasons why Jane wants to make diet changes. This is a very important step. The reason to change needs to out-weigh any of the barriers, and it will help keep the patient on the path to achieving a goal.

Review of the Goal-Setting Process

To review, here are the steps to use to help patients leave with an achievable and believable action plan:

1. Start your session with a patient with a question such as, "What is your biggest concern today?"
2. Guide your patient with open-ended questions, like "Tell me more . . . ."
3. Use reflective listening—paraphrase and repeat back to the patient what she just told you.
4. Identify a change that is important to the patient, something she wants to do.
5. Next make sure she leaves with an action plan based on the WHAT system.
6. Before the session ends, check the patient's confidence level on a scale of 0 to 10 (zero means there is no way that the patient feels she can accomplish the goal and 10 means she is absolutely certain that she will be successful). You want your patient to have a confidence level of at least 7. If her confidence level is lower, guide the person toward revising the goal to make it more achievable (6).
7. Arrange follow-up—it may be via e-mail, phone call, fax, or appointment within the next 2 weeks.

Jane's Story: Part 3

Let's work through another example with Jane. She wants to lose weight, and her RD, Kate, aims to help her set a behavior goal that allows her to work toward her ultimate goal of weight loss. Remember, Jane needs to determine what she wants to work on. For weight loss, her goal will probably be linked to eating, drinking, or physical activity.

> **Kate:** Jane, you said you are concerned about your weight. You are upset with the 30 pounds you gained over the past 2 years, and you just mentioned that your doctor

told you that the health problems you are having are linked to your weight gain. You told me your blood pressure is too high, and you now need two types of medications to control it. You also said that your blood sugar and cholesterol are going up. What is the one thing you want to do this week that will help you with your goal to lose weight and ultimately improve your health?

Jane: I need to change my eating habits.

Kate: What is one thing you want to do differently this week regarding your eating habits?

Jane: I eat too much after dinner.

Kate: It sounds like you want to eat less after dinner.

Jane: Yes—I want to stop eating snacks after dinner.

Kate: Okay, so your main focus will be not eating snacks after dinner. *(Note: Following the WHAT system, this first part of the discussion answers the questions of **what** Jane wants to do and **when** she wants to do it. Therefore, Kate moves on to **how often** Jane wants to skip evening snacks. Kate already set the **time frame** at 1 week.)* How many nights this week do you want to stop snacking?

Jane: Every night. I don't want to eat evening snacks at all. *(Note: When a patient reaches this point of defining a specific goal, you will want to check her confidence level.)*

Kate: Jane, on a scale of 0 to 10, zero being there is no way you can go without after-dinner snacks every day to 10 being absolutely certain you can skip after-dinner snacks every day, where are you? *(Note: It may be helpful to have a scale similar to Figure 6.1 for patients to use when setting their confidence level.)*

Jane: I think I'm at about 5. *(Note: Hearing this number, Kate sets out to do a little probing. She needs to help Jane increase her confidence level.)*

Kate: How many times a week do you have a snack after dinner?

Jane: Every night. *(Note: Going "cold turkey" seems like it is going to be too difficult for Jane. Often, setting a goal for three to five times a week is more realistic, but let your patient make that decision.)*

Kate: What changes could you make to your goal so your confidence level goes up to at least 7?

Jane: If I started with no snacks two times a week and had something healthy for a snack twice a week, then I would be at a 7.

Kate: Okay, for part of your goal, I hear that you want to go snack-free for 2 nights this week. Which evenings would you like to choose?

Jane: I take a pottery class on Monday night, so that would be a good night to skip a snack. My husband works late on Wednesday evening. That would be another good night to go snack-free.

Kate: You are choosing to skip your evening snack on Monday and Wednesday. Now, for the other part of your goal, which 2 evenings do you want to have healthier snacks, and what will those snacks be?

Jane: Friday night we go to the movies, so I will just have popcorn at the movie. Then I will have fresh veggies on Tuesday night. *(Note: Listening to Jane, Kate thinks about how many calories and how much fat are in movie popcorn.)*

Kate: May I offer you some suggestions on healthful snacks? *(Note: Kate is "asking for permission" before she offers her expert advice to Jane.)*

Jane: Sure, I need all the help I can get.

Kate: I have a handout here that lists some suggested choices for low-calorie, healthful snacks. You will notice that veggies are on here—great choice! Air-popped popcorn is also on the list. A 3-cup serving is only about 100 calories; you can also pop the corn in the microwave in a bag if you don't have an air popper. On this other handout, it lists some snack comparisons. You will notice that a small buttered popcorn at the movie theater is almost 600 calories. If you get it unbuttered, then is about 350 calories. While popcorn can be a healthy low-calorie choice, you may want to consider how it is prepared, and how much you are going to have.

Jane: Wow. I didn't know movie theater popcorn has that many calories. I think I will skip the popcorn at the movie and make my own on Saturday night. Plus, this will save me some money!

Kate: To sum up, your plan is to be snack-free after dinner on Monday and Wednesday evenings. Then you plan to choose healthy, lower calorie snacks after dinner twice a week—veggies on Tuesday and air-popped popcorn on Saturday night.

Jane: That is correct!!

Kate: Let's check your confidence level again about your new snacking goal for this coming week. The scale starts at zero—as a reminder, that means you are

100% certain that you *cannot* achieve your goal. The other end of the scale is 10. At that end, you are absolutely certain that you *can* reach your goal of changing your snacking for 4 evenings this week. Where would you rate yourself, Jane?

Jane: I am ready to make some changes so that I can lose weight. This doesn't seem like a very hard first step, so I would rate myself at an 8.

Kate: Jane, that's great. You may want to write your goal for this week down and consider posting it somewhere at home, somewhere you would see it often. Also, logging your progress on evening snacking can be helpful.

Jane: That is a good idea. I will write it down right now and put it on my refrigerator when I get home. Then I will write down what I eat and drink every night after dinner.

Kate: The fridge door is where I post things that I want to remember too!! And I also track goals I set for myself. I plan to meet with you a week from today at 2 PM.

Practice Exercises

Exercise 1

Practice helping your patients put the WHAT into their goal setting.

Exercise 2

Take the goal that you wrote down for yourself in Chapter 3, and put it into the WHAT format. Measure your confidence level and revise your goal if you are not at a 7 or higher. Consider setting your action plan for 1 week and track your progress. Write down your plan:

- *What* will you do? *When* will you do it? And *where*?
- *How much* or *how many*? And *how often*?
- Is your plan *achievable* and believable (use the confidence scale)?
- Your *time frame* is 1 week from today!

References

1. Norris SL, Lau J, Smith SJ, Schmid CH, Engelgau MM. Self-management education for adults with type 2 diabetes: a meta-analysis of the effect on glycemic control. *Diabetes Care.* 2002;25:1159–1171.
2. Renders CM, Valk GD, Griffin SJ, Wagner EH, Eijk VJ, Assendelft WJ. Intervention to improve the management of diabetes in primary care, outpatient and community settings: a systematic review. *Diabetes Care.* 2001;24:1821–1833.
3. Polonsky WH, Earles J, Smith S, Pease DJ, Macmillan M, Christensen R, Taylor T, Dickert J, Jackson RA. Integrating medical management

with diabetes self-management training: a randomized control trial of the Diabetes Outpatient Intensive Treatment program. *Diabetes Care.* 2003;26:3048–3053.

4. Brown SA, Blozis SA, Kouzekanani K, Garcia AA, Winchell M, Hanis CL. Dosage effects of diabetes self-management education for Mexican Americans: the Starr County Border Health Initiative. *Diabetes Care.* 2005;28:527–532.

5. Bodenheimer T, Davis C, Holman H. Helping patients adopt healthier behaviors. *Clin Diabetes.* 2007;25:66–70.

6. Lorig K, Sobel D, Gonzalez V, Minor M. *Living a Healthy Life with Chronic Complications.* Boulder, CO: Bull Publishing; 2006.

When Patients Need More
than Nutrition Counseling

As a registered dietitian (RD), you will encounter patients who may or may not be ready to make lifestyle changes. Often, you may not fully understand the reasons why these patients are not open to change. In Chapter 1, we noted that all of us have worked with "noncompliant" patients (ie, patients who do not return for their follow-up appointments regardless of how hard we try to get them back). In Chapters 3 through 6, we explored several techniques to help us engage our patients. We discussed the importance of letting patients set the agenda and working with patients to ensure the goals they set are individualized and based on the lifestyle changes they want to make. Despite your best efforts, however, some patients still do not seem to be ready or able to make changes. What is going on with these patients?

Many health care professionals have experienced the frustration of working with patients who have chronic health care conditions but don't make positive behavior changes. What else do we need to explore to engage these patients? The Diabetes Attitudes, Wishes, and Needs (DAWN) study (1) looked at this question and reached some important conclusions. This international cross-sectional study used questionnaires to explore how patients and health care professionals perceived diabetes and the stressors surrounding this disease. The study included 5,140 people who had either type 1 or type 2 diabetes, as well as 2,705 physicians and 112 nurses. Among the participants, 19.4% of those with type 1 diabetes and 16.2% of those with type 2 diabetes indicated that they followed self-management recommendations set by their health care professionals (1). These results support what we discussed in previous chapters: the choices patients make every day will have a much larger impact on their diabetes and other medical outcomes than any decision the health care provider makes during a medical appointments (2).

The DAWN study also explored the level of distress patients felt during diagnosis, as well as several years after getting the diagnosis. More than 85% of the participants with diabetes reported high distress levels at the time of diagnosis. Even 15 years later, participants indicated that their treatment was too complicated, and one third stated they were tired of taking their medication. On the other hand, the study showed that many of the health care professionals were frustrated their patients did not follow their advice. They believed that many of their patients were not achieving desirable health outcomes and were experiencing devastating complications as a result of their noncompliance with recommended health care treatment (1).

The results from the DAWN study are changing the way we work with individuals who have diabetes. Much more emphasis is being placed on the emotional distress experienced by our patients. A simple question—"What concerns you the most about your diabetes?"—helps the health care professional explore that emotional distress (3). Patient responses give us an insight into what is really bothering our patients and helps us determine whether they are ready to make lifestyle changes. When we ask this question, we might learn that a patient has difficulty adapting to or accepting the disease, family or work issues, or financial stressors. Many patients who are working on their lifestyle changes could increase their success level if they also received appropriate emotional support from their family, friends, health care team, and others. Other patients may have mental health concerns, such as depression or anxiety, that make it difficult for them to focus on their health. In addition to affecting self-care, untreated mental health disorders can negatively affect relationships and job performance and elevate stress levels. Living with a mental health issue is also linked with increased alcohol and drug use and more difficultly following medical regimens (4).

RDs can play a very important role in identifying these concerns. When working with patients who have chronic diseases, we need to be prepared to identify potential mental health concerns and make the appropriate referrals. In this chapter, we discuss some of these conditions and explore assessment tools that will be helpful in your decision making. This chapter also provides ways to help patients whose self-management and health care are affected by financial constraints.

Mental and Emotional Health Issues

A report of the US Surgeon General estimates that one in five Americans experiences some type of mental health illness in any given year, and two out of three people with mental illness will not seek help (4). According to Sederer and associates (5), there is "overwhelming evidence that mental disorders and medical illnesses are strongly linked." They continue:

> Medical illnesses such as cardiovascular disease, diabetes, asthma, and cancer are associated with mental illnesses, and the more serious the medical condition, the more likely it is that the patient will experience a mental illness. Individuals with depressive disorders are about twice as likely to develop coronary artery disease, twice as likely to have a stroke, more than four times as likely to have a myocardial infarction (MI), and four times as likely to die within 6 months of an MI as people without depressive disorders. Depression is a common poststroke condition, and effective treatment of depression can improve cognitive functioning and survival. People with diabetes are two times as likely to have depression as the general population, and the presence of depression as a comorbidity to diabetes is associated with poor adherence to medication regimens, greater complications of diabetes, increased numbers of emergency room visits, and poorer physical and mental functioning.

Clearly, the detection of possible mental health issues and appropriate referrals are very important. Have a plan in place to help patients who may have a mental illness. Set up lines of communication with the primary care providers so you can closely coordinate your efforts to identify patients' mental health concerns. For example, determine whether mental health screening will be a part of the primary care visit and/or explored by you.

Whether or not you screen patients, you should communicate any concerns about their mental health to the primary care practitioner. Addressing mental health concerns is a key step for your patients to achieve success when making lifestyle changes to maintain or improve their health outcomes.

One strategy to assist patients is to make available educational materials about stress, depression, and anxiety, and where to get additional help. These materials increase awareness about the topics and enable your patients to know they can broach the topic with you (6).

Depression

Since depression can be a common problem, especially for people with chronic health conditions, it is recommended that you have a plan in place for depression screening. Working with primary care providers is essential. Learn whether they regularly screen patients for depression. If they do, do you have access to the results of the assessment and the treatment plan?

If the primary care team does not routinely screen patients, determine how you can work together with the provider to develop a process for including depression screening as part of patient care. This process may include screening patients who concern you and referring them back to their primary care providers for a more detailed assessment and care. Another option may be to help the primary care offices develop and implement a plan to detect and treat depression in the clinics. This process may also require that this information be shared with you during the referral process.

The Patient Health Questionnaire PHQ-2 and PHQ-9 are two tools used for depression screening (7). The PHQ-2 (Figure 7.1) asks just two questions and is easy and quick to administer in any setting. It lets the RD (or other health care provider) determine which patients would benefit from a more in-depth depression

---

PHQ-2 Questionnaire for Major Depressive Disorders

During the past month:

Have you often been bothered by feeling down, depressed, or hopeless?

☐ Yes ☐ No

Have you often been bothered by little interest or pleasure in doing things?

☐ Yes ☐ No

NOTE: An affirmative answer to either question is a positive test result; a negative answer to both questions is a negative test result.

FIGURE 7.1 PHQ-2 Questionnaire for Major Depressive Disorders. Reprinted with permission from Pfizer. All rights reserved.

---

assessment and treatment, which is done or coordinated by the primary care provider. A "yes" answer to one or both of the questions on the PHQ-2 is considered a positive response and indicates that a person may have depression. However, it is not a perfect tool. Research indicates that this sort of quick screen may provide five false positives for every accurate positive response (8). In addition, the PHQ-2 is best for identifying major depressive disorders and does not enable a practitioner to measure the impact of a person's depression on activities of daily living. A positive initial screen should be followed with more in-depth screening by a physician using a detailed tool like the PHQ-9 (Figure 7.2) (7).

Nine-Symptom Depression Checklist
Patient Health Questionnaire (PHQ-9)

Patient Name: _____

Date: _____

Over the *last 2 weeks*, how often have you been bothered by any of the following problems?

		Not at all	Several days	More than half the days	Nearly every day
1.	Little interest or pleasure in doing things.	☐	☐	☐	☐
2.	Feeling down, depressed, or hopeless.	☐	☐	☐	☐
3.	Trouble falling/staying asleep, sleeping too much.	☐	☐	☐	☐
4.	Feeling tired or having little energy.	☐	☐	☐	☐
5.	Poor appetite or overeating.	☐	☐	☐	☐
6.	Feeling bad about yourself or that you are a failure or have let yourself or your family down.	☐	☐	☐	☐
7.	Trouble concentrating on things, such as reading the newspaper or watching television.	☐	☐	☐	☐
8.	Moving or speaking so slowly that other people could have noticed. Or the opposite: being so fidgety or restless that you have been moving around a lot more than usual.	☐	☐	☐	☐
9.	Thoughts that you would be better off dead or of hurting yourself in some way.	☐	☐	☐	☐

FIGURE 7.2 PHQ-9: Nine-Symptom Depression Checklist. Reprinted with permission by Pfizer. *(continues)*

PHQ-9* Questionnaire for Depression Scoring and Interpretation Guide
For physician use only

Scoring: Count the number (#) of boxes checked in a column. Multiply that number by the value indicated below, then add the subtotal to produce a total score. The possible range is 0-27. Use the table below to interpret the PHQ-9 score.

Not at all	(#) _____	× 0	=	_____
Several days	(#) _____	× 1	=	_____
More than half the days	(#) _____	× 2	=	_____
Nearly every day	(#) _____	× 3	=	_____
Total score:				_____

Interpreting PHQ-9 Scores

Diagnosis	Total Score
Minimal depression	0–4
Mild depression	5–9
Moderate depression	10–14
Moderately severe depression	15–19
Severe depression	20–27

Action for Score

≤ 4   The score suggests the patient may not need depression treatment.

5–14 Physician uses clinical judgment about treatment, based on patient's duration of symptoms and functional impairment.

> 14 Warrants treatment for depression, using antidepressants, psychotherapy and/or a combination of treatment.

FIGURE 7.2 *(continued)*
*PHQ-9 is described in more detail at the McArthur Institute on Depression & Primary Care Web site: www.depression-primarycare.org/clinicians/toolkits/materials/forms/phq9.

This helps the physician diagnose, treat, and monitor the severity of depression.

Physicians and mental health professionals may also use other tools, such as the 21-question Beck Depression Inventory, to detect and measure the severity of depression. Additional depression screening tools currently in use include the Medical Outcomes Study Short Form (SF 20) and the Zung Self Rating Depression Scale, which is also available under different names (9). These tools take more time to administer and may require more expertise in the field of depression than an RD typically has.

A depression self-assessment method suggested by Lorig and colleagues in *Living a Healthy Life with Chronic Conditions* is for the patient to ask himself/herself what he/she does to have fun. If the person is unable to answer the question quickly, suspect that depression may be an issue for that person (10).

If you are going to play a role in depression screening and you suspect a patient may have depression, you may broach the subject by mentioning to your patient, "Sometimes people have a lot of extra stress in their lives that may make it difficult to make healthful changes. This stress can be linked to having health problems, job or family issues, or financial concerns. When that is the case, extra help and sometimes medications can help people cope. I have a fast and simple screening tool [eg, a self-assessment version of the PHQ-9] that can help identify whether a person would benefit from additional help or medication. I can help you go through it right now, if you are interested, or I can give you a copy to take home and look over. What would you like to do?" If the patient decides to take the tool home, recommend that she let you or her physician know what the assessment showed.

Ideally, the primary care practitioner takes the lead in the depression diagnosis and treatment. Current guidelines suggest the physician schedule a full diagnostic interview with a patient who has a positive depression screening (11). In addition, the provider may also want to assess thyroid function, vitamin B-12 deficiency, sleep disorders, liver function, and other possible medical causes for signs of depression.

As we mentioned earlier in this chapter, if the primary care practitioner has not screened the patient for depression or if you suspect the patient may have a depression problem, it is appropriate for you to screen the patient. Referring the patient back to their practitioner and following up with the practitioner is crucial to make sure the patient is receiving a more detailed assessment and care, if indicated.

When patients are screened for depression, it is critical to have support services in place (6).

Patients with depressive disorders have successfully responded to short-term psychotherapy, with or without the addition of medication. Be prepared to reinforce medication regimens and discuss nutrition-related issues. For example, if medication is used, the patient will typically not see any effects on their mood for 2 to 6 weeks. However, patients often expect immediate results and may be disappointed if they do not know what will happen. If medications are prescribed, patients will also need to know that they should not stop their depression medication once they feel better. Stopping depression medication abruptly can worsen the symptoms. As an RD, you can work with patients to remind them of this information and check to see whether they are using medications as prescribed. You may also be able to help patients with regular physical activity and stress reduction techniques that are helpful in the management of depression (8). In addition, some medications used to treat depression can affect appetite and weight status, and at least one drug should not be taken with certain foods. Your patients will benefit from knowledge of these drug-nutrient interactions.

Anxiety Disorders

Nearly one quarter of the population will be affected by an anxiety disorder at some time in their lives (12). Anxiety disorders include panic disorder, agoraphobia, obsessive-compulsive disorder, and posttraumatic stress disorder. An overview of these and other types of panic disorders that tend to overwhelm patients and negatively affect their lives can be found on the Freedom from Fear Web site (www.freedomfromfear.org).

Many anxiety disorders are difficult to treat, as patients with anxiety disorders may also have alcoholism, depression, or suicidal thoughts. However, effectively dealing with anxiety disorders can also help with problems that patients have with substance abuse and depression (12).

Anxiety is more common in people with eating disorders than in the general population. Individuals may experience anxiety before their eating disorder developed; anxiety may have even been present during childhood. (Eating disorders are discussed in greater detail later in this chapter.)

To identify anxiety in patients, you could ask as part of the assessment, "What concerns do you have about your condition?" If a patient has diabetes, you could suggest, "Tell me about the aspects of diabetes you worry about" (13). You could also use the GAD7 tool to screen for anxiety. A self-assessment version for patients is posted on the Patient.Co.UK Web site (www.patient.co.uk; from the Home page, search "GAD7") (14). Patients can also go to the

Freedom from Fear Web site (www.freedomfromfear.org) and take an online screening test for anxiety or depression.

Health Distress

Another measure that may be useful, especially among your patients who have serious health conditions, is a measurement of health distress. Figure 7.3 shows a tool, called the Health Distress Scale, which Lorig and colleagues at Stanford University (15) adopted from the Medical Health Outcome Study (16). This tool can give you an idea of how much distress patients are feeling related to their illnesses or health conditions. Like depression or anxiety, patients may need additional treatment for health distress before they are able to effectively implement positive self-management strategies.

Eating Disorders

It is crucial to identify when a patient has a disordered eating condition and make referrals for additional assistance as indicated. The major classifications of eating disorders include (17):

- Anorexia nervosa: the patient has an excessive self-push to become thin. Most will maintain a low body weight and show a deep level of concern with weight gain.
- Bulimia nervosa: the person does not seem to be able to control eating. Most overeat and then vomit, take laxatives, or exercise excessively. People with bulimia also show an exaggerated concern for being overweight.
- Other eating disorders: there are additional eating disorders that do not meet the criteria for anorexia or bulimia;

These questions are about how you feel and how things have been with you during the past month. For each question in the chart below, please circle the **one** number that comes closest to the way you have been feeling.

How much time during the past month . . .	None of the time	A little of the time	Some of the time	A good bit of the time	Most of the time	All of the time
1. Were you discouraged by your health problems?	0	1	2	3	4	5
2. Were you fearful about your future health?	0	1	2	3	4	5
3. Was your health a worry in your life?	0	1	2	3	4	5
4. Were you frustrated by your health problems?	0	1	2	3	4	5

Scoring: Score each item as the number circled. If two consecutive numbers are circled [for an item], score the higher (more distress) number. If the numbers [circled for an item] are not consecutive, do not score the item. The scale score is the mean of the four items. If more than one item is missing, set the value of the scale to missing. Scores range from 0 to 5; higher scores indicate more distress about health.

FIGURE 7.3 Health distress scale used by Lorig and colleagues (15). Adapted with permission from Stewart AL, Hays RD, Ware JE, Health perceptions, energy/fatigue, and health distress measures. In Stewart AL, Ware JE. *Measuring Functioning and Well Being: The Medical Outcomes Study Approach.* Durham NC: Duke University; Press:143–172.

they are referred to as eating disorders not otherwise specified (EDNOS).

The prevalence of eating disorders is unknown, as many people are secretive about their disordered eating. Young women between the ages of 18 and 30 years seem to be the group most affected by disordered eating. Men can also have eating disorders, with gay men having a potentially higher risk than heterosexual men. Athletes (both male and female) also seem to be affected by eating disorders; bulimia is the most common type of eating disorder among athletes. Individuals who want to lose weight and seek help toward this end are the most likely population to have disordered eating. As many as 50% of that group may have an eating disorder (17).

Individuals with an excessive concern about weight and body shape, those with poor self-esteem, and those with a history of sexual abuse or other traumatic experiences are more likely to develop eating disorders (16). In addition, other psychiatric disorders are often linked with eating disorders.

Patients with eating disorders can benefit greatly from the services of a treatment team that includes a mental health specialist as well as an RD. Some patients may need medications to treat the eating disorder or other mental health disorders (such as posttraumatic stress disorder or obsessive-compulsive disorder). Depending on the severity of their eating disorder, some may also benefit from an inpatient program.

Medical nutrition therapy is also an essential component of treatment. In its position statement on nutrition intervention in the treatment of anorexia nervosa, bulimia nervosa, and other eating disorders, the American Dietetic Association reinforces the role of the RD in helping to develop a nutrition plan in coordination with the patient with an eating disorder as well as other team members. Ideally, the RD then establishes an ongoing relationship with the patient to help with the achievement of treatment and nutrition-related goals. When working with patients with eating disorders, RDs will benefit from having enhanced knowledge of behavioral health care (17).

Financial Concerns

Some patients may not share their financial concerns with members of their health care team. For example, they may take less medication than prescribed or be unable to purchase healthful foods because of financial constraints. They may also live in areas with limited local resources, such as grocery stores or pharmacies, or lack means of transportation. Consider asking patients whether money concerns have ever caused them to delay or not follow medical care recommendations. A simple question to ask is, "Do you have trouble paying for . . . ?" Or you could say, "Some of my patients have had trouble paying for some of their medication. Has that happened to you?" If you find that a patient has financial concerns, a referral to a medical social worker may help the person access programs that assist with medical and health care expenses.

You can also provide helpful information to patients on local free or low-cost services. Some of these services might include the following:

- Clinics and hospitals with sliding scales
- Medication assistance programs
- Medicaid programs
- Veteran's Administration programs

- Senior services provided through your area agency on aging or local senior centers
- Organizations specific to certain conditions (eg, Arthritis Foundation, American Diabetes Association, National Kidney Foundation)
- Religious institutions (such as the Catholic Diocese or Lutheran Social Services) and social service organizations
- Local federally qualified health centers
- Health department services
- Food pantries

Recognize your limitations as you seek to assist others—you will not be able to help every person who walks through your door. Sometimes, other health care professionals or different services are a priority for the patient. Do what you can to screen patients and make appropriate referrals to other sources of help. When patients address mental health, family issues, and financial concerns, they often move closer toward being able to work with you on health behavior changes.

Practice Exercises

Exercise 1

Do you and other health care providers with whom you work have a process in place to assess patients for mental health concerns? If yes, what is the process? If not, how can you help put something into place?

Exercise 2

Are adequate resources in place to address mental health conditions in your community? If not, do you have ideas on how your community and health system(s) might enhance services available?

References

1. Funnell M. The Diabetes Attitudes, Wishes, and Needs (DAWN) study. *Clin Diabetes.* 2006;24:154–155.
2. Rubin RR, Anderson RM, Funnell MM. Collaborative diabetes care. *Pract Diabetol.* 2002;21:29–32.
3. Anderson RM, Funnell MM. *Diabetes Concerns Assessment Form.* Ann Arbor, MI: Michigan Diabetes Research and Training Center, University of Michigan; 2005.
4. Office of the US Surgeon General. Mental Health: A Report of the Surgeon General. http://www.surgeongeneral.gov/library/mentalhealth/home.html. Accessed November 14, 2009.
5. Sederer LI, Silver L, McVeigh KH, Levy J. Integrating care for medical and mental illnesses. *Prev Chronic Dis.* 2006;3:A33. http://www.cdc.gov/PCD/issues/2006/apr/05_0214.htm. Accessed November 14, 2009.
6. US Preventive Services Task Force. Screening for Depression in

Adults. http://www.uspreventiveservicestaskforce.org/uspstf09/ adultdepression/addeprrs.htm Accessed October 9, 2010.

7. Ebell MH. Screening instruments for depression. *Am J Family Med.* 2008;78:244–246.

8. Arrol B, Khim N, Kerse N. Screening for depression in primary care with two verbally asked questions: cross sectional study. *BMJ.* 2003;327:1144–1146.

9. Halstenson C, Brunzell C. Depression, celiac disease, and cystic fibrosis. In: Ross T, Boucher J, O'Connell B. *Diabetes Medical Nutrition Therapy and Education.* Chicago, IL: American Dietetic Association; 2005:146–156.

10. Lorig K, Holman H, Sobel D, Laurent D, Gonzalez V, Minor M. *Living a Healthy Life with Chronic Conditions.* 3rd ed. Boulder, CO: Bull Publishing; 2006.

11. Putting prevention into practice: an evidence based approach. *Am Fam Physician.* 2003;67:1561–1562. http://www.aafp.org/ afp/2003/0401/p1561.html. Accessed October 9, 2010.

12. Freedom from Fear Web site. http://www.freedomfromfear.org. Accessed June 12, 2010.

13. American Association of Diabetes Educators. *The Art and Science of Diabetes Self-Management Education: A Desk Reference for Health Care Professionals.* Chicago, IL: American Association of Diabetes Educators; 2006.

14. Generalised Anxiety Disorder Assessment. Patient.co.UK Web site. http://www.patient.co.uk/doctor/Generalised-Anxiety-Disorder-Assessment-(GAD-7).htm. Accessed December 13, 2009.

15. Stanford Patient Education Research Center. Health distress. http:// patienteducation.stanford.edu/research/healthdistress.html. Accessed December 3, 2009.

16. Stewart AL, Hays RD, Ware JE. Health perceptions, energy/fatigue, and health distress measures. In Stewart AL, Ware JE. *Measuring Functioning and Well Being: The Medical Outcomes Study Approach.* Durham NC: Duke University; Press:143–172.

17. Position of the American Dietetic Association: Nutrition intervention in the treatment of anorexia nervosa, bulimia nervosa, and other eating disorders. *J Am Diet Assoc.* 2006;106:2074–2082.

8

Building Long-Term Support for Patients

In the previous chapters, you learned about evidence- and re-
search-based patient counseling techniques, such as empowerment, motivational interviewing, and reflective listening, and explored ways to implement these techniques in your own practice.
At this point, you are better prepared to disarm those surly patients who come in with the attitude of a strong willed 2-year-old
(or teenager or spouse) and are only interested in doing things
their way. (You know the ones—they may sit with their arms
crossed and make statements like, "I don't want to exercise, I
don't want to start eating broccoli, and I am certainly not going to
give up my beer and cigarettes!")

Maybe your patients are not yet doing everything that you
and their other health care providers think they should do to manage their health conditions. Remember, making lifestyle changes
and setting goals is not really about what we believe our patients

should be doing, but what they are willing to change. As long as your patients are doing something positive, that is what counts. When you help them identify the lifestyle changes they want to make and then work with them to develop achievable goals, your patients build self-confidence. By assisting them with problem solving and developing relapse prevention plans, you help them to manage their behavior change over time and in a variety of circumstances. As the old saying goes, success breeds success. How you work with patients on their first goal will set the stage for success or failure with future goals. And the approaches you use *are* helping your patients choose success!

As your patients make lifestyle changes that involve doing things differently, day after day, they will need long-term support. You are part of that support team, but even when you see patients once a week or twice a month, they are still on their own 99% of the time. You won't be with them at the grocery store or when they eat out. You aren't there at 6 AM to get them out of bed for a walk, and you can't police nighttime eating. What are some options for ongoing support?

Options for Ongoing Support

Continued Individual Sessions

You can continue to support patients over the long term through individual meetings, or you can link with them via technology, such as telephone, e-mail, videoconferencing, or Web-based support. You already helped them get to this point. Therefore, you have shown that you have effective clinical and counseling skills. There is every reason to believe that ongoing contact with you will continue to work for your patients. In fact, the American Dietetic Association's Evidence Analysis Library documents the benefits of ongoing interaction with a registered dietitian (RD). Several studies have indicated that the more time people spent with RDs, the more their low-density lipoprotein (LDL) and total cholesterol levels dropped (1). However, questions about long-term support inevitably arise: what methods will you use to provide the support, and how will it be paid for?

RD-Led Group Sessions

Group sessions can be more time- and cost-effective than individual sessions, and they offer the benefit of people learning from and supporting each other. In three studies of group vs individual sessions to target weight loss or diabetes management in middle-aged subjects, the group sessions were *more* effective in the short term than the individual sessions (2–4). More studies are indicated, however.

One of the studies that looked at weight loss in overweight or obese premenopausal women also offered meal replacements in two of the arms of the study (2). All participants attended 26 sessions over a 1-year period. The most successful group was led by an RD and incorporated two meal replacements each day—each participant lost an average of 9.1 pounds. The other arms included an RD-led group with no meal replacement (4.1 pounds lost) and a physician office–based intervention, with meal replacements and individual visits with the doctor and nurse (4.3 pounds lost). Participants in the RD-led group with meal replacement also had significantly more health improvements (lowering of blood pressure, cholesterol, triglycerides, and blood glucose levels) than the other two groups.

A 3-month study in Canada compared individual nutrition counseling with one-on-one sessions that were coupled with group education in adults with type 2 diabetes (4). Participants in the group sessions had significantly greater adherence to nutrition recommendations, identified that they felt like they had more control over their eating, and exhibited a higher level of intention to make diet changes.

Another short-term (3-month) study also looked at weight loss (3). Participants in the group therapy had significantly greater weight loss than those who only participated in the individual counseling.

Peer Support

> *"That we humans can help each other is one*
> *of our unique human capacities."*
> —MARTIN LUTHER KING JR.

People can and do ask for health care–related advice from peers, family members, and even total strangers. One of the authors recently chatted with an employee at a gas station convenience store, who mentioned that a customer with diabetes asked her for advice about which of the store's food items were diabetes-friendly. The employee was not sure what to tell him. After that encounter, she called one of the authors for advice, as she wanted to be able to help future shoppers and not give out any harmful or bad advice. It seems incredible that a person with diabetes would think that a convenience store employee would also be trained to provide expert nutrition advice, but it happens. And with the proliferation of information (or misinformation) on the Internet, even more advice from unlikely or untrained people is available.

Some forms of peer support may be largely unstructured, such as friend-to-friend help offered on an individual basis. Some support groups may also operate with very little structure. It is difficult to judge how helpful these various relationships and groups are, but it seems that some patients might benefit from such support. Some peer programs involve lay health education and support, whereas others do not.

Other peer-mentoring programs are more structured. One example is Alcoholics Anonymous. It involves a 12-step program in which alcoholics offer peer support to one another as they go through the steps. This model has been adapted for other health-related concerns, such as overeating. Some of the more structured peer-led support programs can be effective at helping those with health issues initiate positive behavior change.

The Robert Wood Johnson Foundation has financed a variety of programs to pilot ways to enhance community-based support for people with diabetes. For example, Move More, a free peer-to-peer program in Maine trained lay volunteers to give support to people with type 2 diabetes who desired to get more physically active. Mentees also received pedometers, a nutrition and physical activity guide, and information about indoor and outdoor walking areas. Move More effectively built a network of 40 volunteers who supported people in getting more physically active using a variety of methods (5).

Some diabetes self-management programs have been using *promotoras* (trained lay leaders) to teach diabetes education classes in some Spanish-speaking communities. Another of the Robert Wood Johnson Diabetes Initiatives in Texas evaluated the use of *promotoras* in teaching diabetes classes. They were trained to teach a 10-week series of classes, followed by ten weekly support group meetings and weekly phone follow-up. Patients had improvements in metabolic control that were sustained over time (6).

Another structured program that offers peer support is the Stanford Chronic Disease Self-Management program. Designed to help people with chronic conditions, all potential leaders go through 4 days of training and practice teaching to become certified to lead the program. The program was designed to use lay leaders who also live with chronic health conditions. It is cofacilitated by two trained leaders, and a scripted manual helps guide the leaders through the six workshops that make up this program. One of the basic parts of the program is helping participants set and achieve goals each week. A study that followed 1,000 patients in the program for 3 years showed that participants were more active, reported less health distress, and saved health care dollars (7).

Some weight-loss programs, such as Weight Watchers and TOPS (Take Off Pounds Sensibly), use peers to help and support each other. Tsai and Wadden systematically reviewed the effectiveness of these weight-loss programs and others (8). Unfortunately, the authors were not able to identify many well-designed studies that examined different weight-loss programs. Weight Watchers had the best published data of any of the commercial or e-diet programs. In Weight Watchers, participants lost an estimated 10% of their body weight and were maintaining 3% of that weight loss after 2 years.

Technology Support

> "Getting information off the Internet is like
> taking a drink from a fire hydrant."
>
> —MITCHELL KAPOR

This is the age of technology support, whether it is provided by you, other health care providers, family, friends, individual online peers, or peer support communities. Technological methods of communication include the phone, fax, e-mail, text messaging, instant message, chat, blog, Twitter, Facebook, or other social media. Webinars, DVDs, and videoconferences are other communication vehicles. Some support is also available through automated phone calls or Smartphone applications. Will one or more of these methods be helpful for some of your patients? Will they be part of your services or another totally separate program?

Internet-based weight-loss programs have proliferated; for example, Weight Watchers has an online version. Some are described in more detail in the resources listed in the Appendix. One study recently compared an online weight control program to one that also included weekly behavior counseling e-mails and feedback from a counselor. Participants in both groups were at risk of developing type 2 diabetes and had started the program with a face-to-face meeting. All had the same Internet weight-loss program and all were instructed to submit their weights weekly. Adding the weekly e-mail and feedback to the Internet approach significantly improved weight loss over the yearlong program (4.4 vs 2.0 kg) (9).

Videoconferencing (interactive TV) has been tested as a means of delivering diabetes self-management education. In one study, it was as effective as in-person classes. The videoconference participants rated the classes as helpful as the in-person class participants, and both groups also experienced similar reductions in stress (10).

You have many patients to serve, and helping them identify ways to get continued support with community resources or technology may enable them sustain behavior changes over the long term. Their progress also allows you to move onto helping other patients.

Practice Exercises

Exercise 1

Identify the methods of long-term support you currently offer your patients, and find out about the community support programs that exist in your area. Are there any support groups that your patient population would benefit from?

Exercise 2

To assess what types of ongoing support your patients are receiving and what kinds of outcomes they are achieving, you may want to gather the following information:

a. What percentage of your patients have access to ongoing support?
   i. Do they use these services?
   ii. What type of outcomes do they have? How are you defining/measuring outcomes (eg, through use of clinical data)?
b. Do you have a data-tracking mechanism in place?

Exercise 3

Consider exploring other types of support for your patients, such as reputable Internet chat rooms, video conferencing, or support groups.

References

1. American Dietetic Association Evidence Analysis Library. The relationship between medical nutrition therapy (MNT) by a registered

dietitian and patients' levels of dietary fat, saturated fat, serum cholesterol, and cardiac risk factors. http://www.adaevidencelibrary.com/
evidence.cfm?evidence_summary_id=93. Accessed December 11,
2009.

2. Ashley JM, St. Jeor ST, Schrage JP, Permean-Chaney SE, Gilbertson
MC, McCall NL, Bovee V. Weight control in the physician's office.
Arch Internatl Med. 2001;161:599–604.

3. Renjilian DA, Nezu A, Shermer RL, Perri MG, McKelvey WF, Anton
SD. Individual versus group therapy for obesity: effects of matching
participants to their treatment preferences. *J Consult Clin Psychol.*
2001;69:717–721.

4. Gucciardi E, DeMelo M, Lee R, Grace S. Assessment of two culturally
competent diabetes education methods: individual vs. individual plus
group education in Canadian Portuguese adults with type 2 diabetes.
Ethnic Health. 2007;12:163–187.

5. Richert ML, Webb AJ, Morse NA, O'Toole ML, Brownson CA. Move
More diabetes. *Diabetes Educ.* 2007;33(suppl 6):179S–184S.

6. Joshu CE, Rangel L, Garcia O, Brownson CA, O'Toole ML. Integration of a *promotora*-led self-management program into a system of
care. *Diabetes Educ.* 2007;33(suppl 6):151S–158S.

7. Lorig KR, Ritter P, Stewart AL, Sobel DS, Brown BW, Bandura A,
González VM, Laurent DD, Holman HR. Chronic disease self-
management program: 2-year health status and health care utilization
outcomes. *Med Care.* 2001;39:1217–1223.

8. Tsai AG, Wadden TA. Systematic review: an evaluation of major commercial weight loss programs in the United States. *Ann Intern Med.*
2005;142:56–66.

9. Tate DF, Jackvony EH, Wing RR. Effects of Internet behavioral counseling on weight loss in adults at risk for type 2 diabetes. *JAMA.*
2003;289:1833–1836.

10. Izquierdo RE, Knudson PE, Meyer S, Kearns J, Ploutz-Snyder R,
Weinstock RS. A comparison of diabetes education administered
through telemedicine versus in person diabetes care. *Diabetes Educ.*
2003;26:1002–1007.

Other Issues to Consider: Health Literacy, Cultural Diversity, and Biases in Health Care

In this book, we have discussed how to help patients make lifestyle changes and how various approaches will work in different scenarios. We also discussed certain barriers that you may encounter when working with patients, such as depression and other mental health issues and financial barriers to self-care (see Chapter 7). This chapter addresses selected other issues that you will want to consider when working with patients: health literacy, cultural diversity, and various biases, such as age or gender.

Health Literacy

Many of your patients may have low health literacy, and you might not even be aware of it! Health literacy is defined in *Health People 2010* as "The degree to which individuals have the capacity to obtain, process, and understand basic health information and services needed to make appropriate health decisions." Health literacy is more than a person's reading level. It also involves the ability to make what can be complex decisions based on what is read (1). In fact, having low health literacy has been described as a silent epidemic—you can't always discover it just by looking at or talking with a person. Low health literacy can be found in patients of all income levels and across all races, ages, and backgrounds. According to the Institute of Medicine's report *Health Literacy: A Prescription to End Confusion,* nearly 50% of the US population has problems with health literacy, which lead to missed medical appointments, not taking prescriptions as directed, and misunderstanding other medical treatment (2). According to the American Medical Association, low health literacy is "a stronger predictor of a person's health than age, income, employment status, education level, and race" (3).

Health literacy challenges may explain why some patients do not "comply" with certain requirements like reading food labels, following meal plans, taking medications, and filling out insurance forms. As you work to empower your patients, keep in mind that low health literacy may hinder their abilities to take charge of their health care (2).

People with low health literacy are more likely to have chronic health conditions like diabetes, high blood pressure, or HIV/AIDS, and they manage them less effectively than people with higher health literacy levels. In addition, they use more high-cost services to treat health conditions, like emergency room visits and hospitalizations, and they use fewer preventive health services such as flu shots and mammograms (3).

Some US health care professionals mistakenly think health literacy mainly affects people who do not speak English or for whom English is a second language. In reality, only 15% of those who have limited health literacy were born outside the United States (2). While non-native English speakers are at high risk for having low health literacy, so are older adults, people with low incomes, those who did not graduate high school, and racial and ethnic minorities (4).

You may not immediately recognize that someone has limited health literacy, as people can develop ways to hide that they do not understand spoken directions or written materials (particularly if they feel ashamed or embarrassed about their literacy skills) (2). Fortunately, you can adopt a variety of techniques that will enhance your ability to communicate with patients who have health literacy concerns—remember, low health literacy is common! Keep in mind the following when working with a patient who has low health literacy:

- Speak slowly.
- Dump the medical terms. Keep your message simple. (For more help in using plain language, check out the Center for Plain Language Web site: www.centerforplainlanguage .org.)
- Watch for overload. Remember, the patient is in charge. If you want to give advice, ask for permission and offer just a couple of suggestions.
- Check back or "close the loop." Did your patient understand the conversation exchange? Ask person to explain to you what steps they are going to take. Make sure that you do not turn this into a test. Some experts in health literacy suggest that you start with something like, "I want to make certain that I am explaining things well. Taking medications in the right way can be very hard and confusing. Can you please tell me what changes we made in your medications and how you are going to take them?" (5).

- Demonstrate whenever possible and allow patients the opportunity to practice. For example, label reading is a great opportunity to demonstrate and practice with a patient.
- Use handouts that also include pictures. Many studies have indicated that educational handouts and patient consent forms are difficult for many patients to read and comprehend. Recent research has indicated that Internet-based educational materials are also too difficult for many patients. Box 9.1 gives an overview on how to identify or develop patient forms and educational tools that more fully address health literacy concerns (6).

BOX 9.1 *Developing Patient-Friendly Handouts*

- Limit information to one or two educational messages.
- Only cover items patients really need to know.
- Keep content at or below 6th grade reading level (SMOG or FRY are two examples of readability tests you can use to check level).
- Use one- or two-syllable words.
- Avoid medical or dietetics jargon.
- Use a large font (at least 12 point) with upper- and lower-case letters.
- Make certain handout has ample white space.
- Bulleted items are generally easier to read than paragraphs.
- Use simple pictures that are relevant to the topic.

Screening for Health Literacy

Some health care professionals believe that testing for health literacy may be demeaning to patients and prefer to use simple tools and words when working with *all* patients. However, others think that it may be helpful for one of the health care team members to assess each patient's health literacy (2). Work with your health care partners to put in place a plan of action for your team. Will someone screen for health literacy? Will you play a role in screening?

Two reliable and easy-to-use tools that are used to evaluate health literacy are the rapid estimate of adult literacy in medicine (REALM) and the test of functional health literacy (TOFHLA). With REALM, you provide a patient with a list of medical terms that are single syllable (eg, pill, stress) and multiple syllables (eg, inflammatory, potassium), and ask her to read the list. The test takes less than 5 minutes to administer and score. The number of words that a person pronounces correctly helps identify her reading level. In addition, the test helps highlight some of the things the person may need help with, such as reading and following the directions on a prescription label (2).

TOFHLA is a two-part test that is available in English or Spanish. It poses a scenario for participants and then asks them to answer questions about the scenario. They are asked to fill in blank spaces from a multiple-choice list of answers. In addition to being a reading test, TOFHLA also poses numeracy questions, like figuring out how much medication to take and when to take it, based on looking at a drug label.

The Newest Vital Sign (NVS) is a quick and easy health literacy tool available in Spanish and English, which was designed for primary care (7). Patients are given a health scenario and are then verbally asked a series of six questions. The entire screening can take less than 3 minutes. If a person answers four or more of the questions correctly, she probably does not have low health literacy. If she answers fewer than four questions correctly, literacy issues are probably a concern. One NVS scenario of interest to registered dietitians (RDs) is a nutrition label scenario that requires people to do mathematical calculations (see Figures 9.1 and 9.2).

Nutrition Facts

Serving Size	½ cup
Servings per container	4

Amount per serving

Calories	250	Fat Cal	120

	%DV
Total Fat 13g	20%
Sat Fat 9g	40%
Cholesterol 28mg	12%
Sodium 55mg	2%
Total Carbohydrate 30g	12%
Dietary Fiber 2g	
Sugars 23g	
Protein 4g	8%

*Percentage Daily Values (DV) are based on a 2,000 calorie diet. Your daily values may be higher or lower depending on your calorie needs.

Ingredients: Cream, Skim Milk, Liquid Sugar, Water, Egg Yolks, Brown Sugar, Milkfat, Peanut Oil, Sugar, Butter, Salt, Carrageenan, Vanilla Extract.

FIGURE 9.1 Newest Vital Sign Nutrition Label. Newest Vital Sign is copyrighted by Pfizer Inc. and used with permission.

Score Sheet for the Newest Vital Sign Questions and Answers

READ TO SUBJECT: This information is on the back of a container of a pint of ice cream.

	Answer correct?	
	yes	no

1. If you eat the entire container, how many calories will you eat?

   Answer: *1,000 is the only correct answer.*

2. If you are allowed to eat 60 grams of carbohydrates as a snack, how much ice cream could you have?

   Answer: *Any of the following is correct: 1 cup (or any amount up to 1 cup), half the container. Note: If patient answers "two servings," ask "How much ice cream would that be if you were to measure it into a bowl?"*

3. Your doctor advises you to reduce the amount of saturated fat in your diet. You usually have 42 g of saturated fat each day, which includes one serving of ice cream. If you stop eating ice cream, how many grams of saturated fat would you be consuming each day?

   Answer: *33 is the only correct answer.*

4. If you usually eat 2500 calories in a day, what percentage of your daily value of calories will you be eating if you eat one serving?

   Answer: *10% is the only correct answer.*

READ TO SUBJECT: Pretend that you are allergic to the following substances: Penicillin, peanuts, latex gloves, and bee stings.

5. Is it safe for you to eat this ice cream?

   Answer: *No.*

6. (Ask only if the patient responds "no" to question 5): Why not?

   Answer: *Because it has peanut oil.*

Number of correct answers:

Interpretation

Score of 0–1 suggests high likelihood (50% or more) of limited literacy.
Score of 2–3 indicates the possibility of limited literacy.
Score of 4–6 almost always indicates adequate literacy.

FIGURE 9.2 Score Sheet for the Newest Vital Sign. Newest Vital Sign is copyrighted by Pfizer Inc. and used with permission.

Additional Health Literacy Resources

In addition to the Center for Plain Language Web site (www
.centerforplainlanguage.org), which we mentioned earlier in this
chapter, there are many other excellent free or low-cost opportunities to improve your health literacy skills. For example, the US
Department of Health and Human Services offers free online
training courses in health literacy (http://www.hrsa.gov/health
literacy/default.htm).

To find more information on developing low-literacy print
materials, visit the Clear and Simple section of the National Cancer Institute Web site (http://www.nci.nih.gov/aboutnci/oc/
clear-and-simple/page1). Also, visit the Web site for the Pharmacy Health Literacy Center (http://pharmacyhealthliteracy
.ahrq.gov/sites/PharmHealthLiteracy/default.aspx), developed by
the Agency for Healthcare Research and Quality. You may get
some useful tips in helping patients understand how and why to
take medications.

Other resources you may want to check out regarding health
literacy include the Institute of Medicine book *Health Literacy:
A Prescription to End Confusion* (2), and the Pfizer Clear Health
Communication Initiative (www.pfizerhealthliteracy.com).

Cultural and Ethnic Diversity

In earlier chapters, we discussed ways to identify patient priorities and use approaches like empowerment and motivational interviewing to help them refine goals. Having knowledge about
and acceptance of food habits and the cultural beliefs of your clients can also be very important in building rapport and helping
your patients set and make behavior changes.

When working with patients, learn about their cultural and ethnic backgrounds. Strive to understand and embrace cultural diversity. The following are some questions to consider as you work with patients from cultures different than yours (2):

- Are there accepted gender norms, such as distinctive roles for men and women?
- Do extended family members play important roles in the patient's life or care?
- What traditional medicine beliefs or practices does the person embrace?
- What foods are accepted, celebrated, or forbidden?
- Do you need to consider culturally specific factors in counseling situations, like the appropriateness of eye contact or touching or the significance of body language?
- What are acceptable styles of dress?

As you consider these issues, remember to assess your patients as individuals—don't jump to conclusions about a specific patient's cultural practices based on general knowledge of that culture. Instead, ask culturally sensitive questions and observe personal behavior.

Use of Translators and Lay Health Workers

Depending on language skills, you may need to have a trained interpreter present to assist with medical terminology and concepts during discussions with your patients. For some patients, having lay health workers involved in care will also be valuable.

Additional Resources on Cultural Diversity

The American Dietetic Association (ADA) has a variety of resources that can help you work with clients who may come from different cultural backgrounds. For example, the book *Culturally Competent Dietetics: Increasing Awareness, Improving Care* is a collection of articles that were previously published in the *Journal of the American Dietetic Association*. It offers practical advice from experts on ways to interact with people from other cultures. *Spanish for the Nutrition Professional*, Second Edition, explores cross-cultural communication techniques, teaches basic counseling phrases and vocabulary, and includes food pictures with their English and Spanish names. You can purchase these books and review other resources on the American Dietetic Association Web site (www.eatright.org).

Identifying and Addressing Biases

One of the authors has a 72-year-old friend, Mary. Recently, Mary went to a sporting goods store to purchase a new pair of racing cross-country skis. Despite her spry physical condition and ability to tell the shop salesperson what she wanted, the clerk, according to Mary, tried to steer her away from the racing skis. Mary felt this was a prime case of age discrimination. If the store clerk had gone out on the trails with Mary, he would have seen that her stamina and skill level were perfectly suited for racing skis. In the end, he did not deter Mary from buying the racing skis either!

Mary persevered in her goals despite the clerk's apparent bias. However, in health care, practitioner biases can have notable consequences for the quality of care that patients receive. Although we all wish to consider ourselves personally free of bias, it is advisable to periodically reflect on these issues and how your perceptions of patients may be shaped by your assumptions about factors such as age, gender, weight, race, or ethnicity.

Age and Gender Bias

Age and gender discrimination have been documented in health care. A UK study involving more than 15,500 people who had been diagnosed with ischemic heart disease found that women, especially women older than age 65 years, were not prescribed the recommended treatment at the same level received by men (8). Another study used a series of videotaped vignettes to "test" how 256 primary care doctors (men and women) would care for different patients. The study participants were similar in age, class, and race. Some of the cases were presented as women and some as men. The biggest difference in treatment was linked to gender. Women across all scenarios were asked fewer questions, received fewer tests, and had fewer medications prescribed (9).

Weight Bias

People with overweight or obesity may be subjected to bias or discriminatory health care practices. One study (10) examined potential weight bias in health care professionals who specialized in the management of obesity and concluded that these health care professionals exhibited a significant "anti-fat" bias. In addition, the health care professionals endorsed the stereotypes of overweight and obese patients being "lazy, stupid, and worthless." Finding bias in this group of health care professionals was particularly surprising, as they understand the complexities of being obese and realize it cannot be simply attributed to personal

choices. Similar weight bias against overweight and obese patients has been identified in other health care professionals, too.
Some have said they spend less time with obese patients and tend
to order more tests. Others have stated they are repulsed by obese
people and would prefer not to treat them (10).

Obese women are less likely to obtain preventive services
such as breast and pelvic exams, even though they see their physicians more often. In part, this is linked to the negative body image
of many obese women and their reluctance to have their bodies
examined. However, some health care providers do not encourage obese women to receive care, and some do not want to examine them (10).

Racial and Ethnic Disparities and Biases

Racial and ethnic differences in health care have been reported.
Several studies have indicated that much of the difference in care
for racial and ethnic minorities is due to socioeconomic factors
and insurance status. Those without insurance, who also tend to
have a lower income, receive fewer medical services. When there
are language barriers, care received is even more suboptimal (11).

Additional Resources to Assess Potential Biases

Project Implicit has online mini assessments (Implicit Association Tests) on a variety of topics to help individuals and researchers look at conscious and unconscious preferences or biases for
more than 90 different issues. Originally launched by Yale University as a demonstration Web site in 1998, Project Implicit has since
grown into a research project overseen by four universities. It has
been funded by the National Institute of Mental Health since 2003.
It has multiple Web sites, including the following:

- ProjectImplicit.net (www.projectimplicit.net), which offers a general overview, news, and links to the other sites.
- The Demonstration section at https://implicit.harvard. edu/implicit, which allows you to complete one or more of the assessments. Each assessment takes about 10 to 15 minutes. At the end of each assessment, participants are given feedback on preferences and potential biases.

Practice Exercises

Exercise 1

How does your practice address health literacy? What about the health care providers and systems you work with? Consider the following questions:

- Are your forms and educational tools patient friendly?
- Do you use teach-back skills and plain language and avoid patient overload?

If you answered "no" to these questions, what is one thing that you can begin implementing?

Exercise 2

What type of cultures or ethnic groups do you work with? If you have not already done so, consider taking time to learn more about their beliefs and practices, especially as linked to health and food.

References

1. Glassman P. Health Literacy. National Network of Libraries of Medicine. http://nnlm.gov/outreach/consumer/hlthlit.html. Accessed February 6, 2011.
2. Institute of Medicine; Nielsen-Bohlman L, Panzer AM, Kindig DA, eds. *Health Literacy A Prescription to End Confusion*. Washington, DC: National Academies Press; 2004. http://books.nap.edu/openbook .php?record_id=10883. Accessed June 27, 2010.

3. Health literacy: report of the Council of Scientific Affairs. Ad Hoc Committee on Health Literacy for the Council on Scientific Affairs, American Medical Association. *JAMA.* 1999;281:552–557.

4. Quick Guide to Health Literacy. US Department of Health and Human Services. http://www.health.gov/communication/literacy/ quickguide/factsliteracy.htm. Accessed November 20, 2009.

5. Schillinger D, Piette J, Grumbach K, et al. Closing the loop: physician communication with diabetic patients who have low health literacy. *Arch Intern Med.* 2003;163:83–90.

6. Weiss BD. Health Literacy and Patient Safety: Help Patients Understand. Manual for Clinicians. American Medical Association Foundation and American Medical Association; 2007. http://www.ama-assn.org/ama1/pub/upload/mm/367/healthlitclinicians.pdf. Accessed May 3, 2011.

7. Weiss BD, May MZ, Martz W, Castro KM, DeWalt DA, Pignone MP, Mockbee J, Hale FA. Quick assessment of literacy in primary care: the newest vital sign. *Ann Family Med.* 2005;3:514–522. http://www.annfammed.org/cgi/reprint/3/6/514. Accessed November 20, 2009.

8. Williams D, Bennett K, Feely J. Evidence for an age and gender bias in the secondary prevention of ischaemic heart disease in primary care. *Br J Clin Pharmacol.* 2003;55:604–608.

9. Arber S, McKinlay J, Adams A, Marceau L, O'Donnell A. Patient characteristics and inequalities in doctors' diagnostic and management strategies relating to CHD: a video-simulation experiment. *Soc Sci Med.* 2006;62:103–115.

10. Schwartz B, Chambliss HO, Brownell KD, Blair SN, Billington C. Weight bias among health professionals specializing in obesity. *Obes Res.* 2003;11:1033–1039.

11. Kirby JB, Taliaferro G, Zuvekas SH. Explaining racial and ethnic disparities in health care. *Med Care.* 2006;44:5.I64–I72.

Appendix

Resources

Chapter 2

Committee on Quality of Health Care in America, Institute of Medicine. *Crossing the Quality Chasm: A New Health System for the 21st Century*. Washington, DC: National Academies Press; 2001. http://books.nap.edu/openbook.php?record_id=10027.

Improving Chronic Illness Care. www.improvingchroniccare.org. Includes access to the Chronic Care Model.

National Diabetes Education Program. Making Systems Changes for Better Diabetes Care. http://betterdiabetescare.nih.gov.

Chapter 3

Anderson B, Funnel M. *The Art of Empowerment: Stories and Strategies for Diabetes Educator*. 2nd ed. Arlington, VA: Skelly

Publishing; 2005. Order from the publisher (www.skelly
publishing.com) or Amazon.com. Available for 30 CPEs until
10/1/2013.

Michigan Diabetes Research and Training Center. www.med
.umich.edu/mdrtc. Offers many books and tools on empowerment. One particularly useful tool is the Diabetes Concerns Assessment Form (www.med.umich.edu/mdrtc/profs/index
.htm#conc). The center also offers a number of survey instruments that can be useful in working with people with diabetes
(www.med.umich.edu/mdrtc/profs/survey.html).

Chapter 4

Prochaska JO, Norcross J, DiClemente C. *Changing for Good: A
Revolutionary Six-Stage Program for Overcoming Bad Habits
and Moving Your Life Positively Forward*. New York, NY: William Morrow and Company; 1994.

Chapter 5

Motivational Interviewing Web site. www.motivationalinterview
.org. Includes motivational training, videos, and resources.

Chapter 6

American Association of Diabetes Educators. AADE®7 System.
www.diabeteseducator.org/ProfessionalResources/AADE7/
A7S.html. Tool to help with patient goal setting and tracking.

Lorig K, Sobel D, Gonzalez V, Minor M. *Living a Healthy Life
with Chronic Complications*. Boulder, CO: Bull Publishing;
2006.

Chapter 7

Mental Health Concerns

American Dietetic Association. Position of the American Dietetic Association: Nutrition intervention in the treatment of anorexia nervosa, bulimia nervosa, and other eating disorders. *J Am Diet Assoc.* 2006;106:2074-2082. www.eatright.org/positions.

Freedom from Fear. www.freedomfromfear.org. Offers depression and anxiety self-assessment tools. Made available by the National Nonprofit Mental Illness Advocacy Organization.

Michigan Diabetes Research and Training Center. Diabetes Concerns Assessment Forms. www.med.umich.edu/mdrtc/ profs/index.htm#conc. Other resources also offered.

Patient Health Questionnaires (PHQ) Screeners. www .phqscreeners.com. Free mental health disorder screening tools available for use by health care professionals. Made available by Pfizer.

Stanford Patient Education Research Center. Health Distress Screening Tool. http://patienteducation.stanford.edu/ research/healthdistress.html.

US Preventive Services Task Force. Recommendation Statement on Screening for Depression in Adults. http://www.uspreventiveservicestaskforce.org/ uspstf09/adultdepression/addeprrs.htm.

Financial Concerns

Local service clubs and churches may also be able to provide short-term assistance, and many health systems also have special programs for patients with financial concerns.

Centers for Medicare & Medicaid Services. Federally Qualified Health Centers (FQHC). https://www.cms.gov/center/fqhc .asp. FQHC provide sliding scale fees for many medical services and medication.

Indian Health Service. www.ihs.gov. Help for American Indians and Alaska Natives.

Needy Meds. www.needymeds.org. Offers help with cost of medication.

Salvation Army. www.salvationarmyusa.org. Offers temporary home, food, and medication assistance.

Senior List. www.SeniorsList.com. Resources for older adults.

Society of Saint Vincent de Paul: http://www.svdpusa.org. Offers temporary home, food, and medication assistance.

US Department of Health and Human Services. www.hhs.gov. Links to health care questions and resources and special insurance for children.

US Department of Veterans Affairs. www.va.gov. Additional help for veterans and widows of veterans. To check eligibility, go to www.va.gov/healtheligibility/Library/tools/Quick_Eligibility_ Check.

Chapter 8

Diabetes Support

Children with Diabetes. www.childrenwithdiabetes.com. Online community for kids, families, and adults with diabetes.

dLife Diabetes Support Forum. www.dlife.com/diabetes-forum. Free forum.

National Diabetes Education Program. Diabetes Health Sense. http://ndep.nih.gov/resources/diabetes-healthsense/index .aspx. Offers resources devoted to supporting patient change, including a searchable database of research, tools, and programs to help you support patient behavior and lifestyle changes.

Kidney Disease Support

DaVita. www.davita.com. Resources and support for those with kidney disease or those on dialysis.

Weight-Loss Support

A partial list; other plans are available.

Calorie King. www.calorieking.com. Food and exercise tracking, online support and resources. Fee charged.

ChooseMyPlate. www.choosemyplate.gov. Resources and interactive tools, including personalized food plans and food tracker. Free.

Diet.com. www.diet.com. Similar to eDiets (described next), but does not have food plan option.

eDiets. www.ediets.com. Provides individualized menus for a variety of meal plans, fitness plans, live phone support, and online communities. Prepackaged food is also available. Fees charged for diet plan, support, and food.

Jenny Craig. www.jennycraig.com. Program includes prepackaged foods. Meeting or phone support available. Fees charged for services.

Nutrisystem. www.nutrisystem.com. For-purchase meal replacement plan with online support.

Overeaters Anonymous. www.oa.org. Support group based on the 12-step program; no fees to attend.

SparkPeople. www.sparkpeople.com. Free weight-loss and fitness Web site; includes food and exercise tracker, questions answered by registered dietitians and fitness experts, links with others who are interested in weight loss, and a variety of resources.

Take Off Pounds Sensibly (TOPS). www.tops.org. Low-cost program that mainly provides support for weight-loss efforts of participants.

Weight Watchers. www.weightwatchers.com. Online or phone and community meetings available. Fees charged for services.

Smart Phone Applications for Weight-Loss Support

Just a small sample of the many apps available; some charge fees.

Concrete Software. Fast Food Calorie Counter (iPhone app). To purchase, go to the iTunes store (www.apple.com/itunes).

Fresh Apps. Lose It! www.freshapps.com/lose-it.

Livestrong.com Calorie Tracker. www.livestrong.com/calorie-counter-mobile.

My Net Diary. www.mynetdiary.com. Includes a calorie counter that allows you to scan food bar codes for nutritional value.

SparkPeople. www.sparkpeople.com/mobile-apps.asp. Free apps available for many smartphones.

Weight Watchers Mobile. Weight Watchers participants can track their points with this iPhone app. To purchase, go to the iTunes store (www.apple.com/itunes).

Chapter 9

Health Literacy Resources for Professionals

Agency for Healthcare Research and Quality. Pharmacy Health Literacy Center. www.ahrq.gov/pharmhealthlit. Resources and information related to health literacy and use of medications.

American Medical Association. Health Literacy Resources. www.ama-assn.org. (search "Health Literacy" from Home page). Offers a manual for clinicians, news, frequently asked questions, and other resources.

Health Resources and Services Administration. Health Literacy. www.hrsa.gov/healthliteracy/default.htm. Free online training courses in health literacy.

National Cancer Institute. Clear and Simple. www.nci.nih.gov/aboutnci/oc/clear-and-simple/page1. Information on developing low literacy print materials.

National Patient Safety Foundation. Ask Me 3. www.npsf.org/askme3. Resources to improve communication with patients who have low health literacy.

The Pfizer Clear Health Communication Initiative. www.pfizerhealthliteracy.com.

Assessment of Bias

Project Implicit. Implicit Association Tests. https://implicit.harvard.edu/implicit. Online mini-assessments on a variety of topics to help individuals and researchers look at conscious and unconscious preferences or biases for more than 90 different issues.

Index

Page number followed by *b* indicates box; *f,* figure; *t,* table.

Index